The BBC Diet

'How long does getting thin take?'
Pooh asked anxiously.
A. A. Milne

THE
BBC DIET

Dr Barry Lynch

BBC Books

The BBC Diet is a healthy way of eating as well as a way of losing weight, but if you are worried about any aspect of your health, check with your doctor before starting on this or any other diet.

Published by BBC Books,
a division of BBC Enterprises Limited
Woodlands, 80 Wood Lane, London W12 0TT
First published 1988
Reprinted 1988, 1989
Second Reprint 1989

© Barry Lynch 1988
ISBN 0 563 20689 6

Set by Wilmaset in 10/11 Sabon
Printed and bound in Great Britain by
Richard Clay Ltd, Bungay, Suffolk
Cover printed by Richard Clay Ltd, Norwich, Norfolk

CONTENTS

This book accompanies the television series *The BBC Diet Programme*, produced by Prospect Pictures for BBC Wales.

ACKNOWLEDGEMENTS

I am grateful – I think! – to Suzanne Webber for persuading me to write this book and for giving me such enthusiastic support during the process. I should also like to thank Teleri Bevan, John Stuart Roberts and John Geraint of BBC Wales for making it possible for me to write it.

Thanks are also due to those who worked so hard on the television series. I am especially grateful to Sarah Brewster, Andy Collie, Pauline Evans, Sarah Ruckley and Tony McAvoy.

I am indebted to Professor John Catford and Helen Howson of Heartbeat Wales for their many valuable suggestions and to Brynda Lewis for her help in assessing the calorie counts of the diet plans.

Anton Mosimann's recipes for barbecued hake kebabs with pink grapefruit (p. 138), crab salad with coconut (p. 142), mixed fish soup with vegetables (p. 134) and sea bass with fresh tomato sauce (p. 137) are reprinted from *Anton Mosimann's Fish Cuisine* (Macmillan) by kind permission.

The diagrams on p. 4 are reproduced from *Diet 2000*, by Dr Alan Maryon-Davis with Jane Thomas, published by Pan Books Ltd.

Finally, my thanks go to Catrin Morgan and Tessa McKenzie who patiently typed the manuscript under great pressure.

CHAPTER 1

INTRODUCTION

If you feel fat, your body is trying to tell you something: lose weight.

I want to assure you that you can get to your ideal weight and stay at your ideal weight – and be and feel healthy – and enjoy food. In fact, you can enjoy as much food as you're eating now: you just need to swap some less-fattening food for some of the fattening food you're eating. Perhaps you're a diet expert, you've tried every one going and your weight has gone up and down like a yo-yo. Or maybe you've never been on a diet before, know you need to lose some weight but are confused by the conflicting advice when you flick through diet books and magazines. Or perhaps you're interested in your family's health and their weight and you want to understand about healthy food as well as slimming food.

Whoever you are, if you let it, this book could change your life. A big claim! A tall story? How do you know I'm not a quack? Well, I am a doctor, but being medically qualified doesn't absolve one from being gullible, stupid or just plain wrong. There are diet books on sale which are written by doctors and are mistaken; in fact they are sometimes shocking in the outdated and incorrect advice they offer.

But the main views expressed in this book, and the principles on which the BBC Diet is based are not only my own: they are also held by the overwhelming majority of medical and nutritional experts in Great Britain and around the world. They have been expressed, confirmed and reiterated over the last decade by over twenty international medical reports and in this country by several reports from DHSS expert committees and the Royal Medical Colleges. There is now a medical consensus on the sort of diet we should follow to lose weight – which is also the most healthy diet we can eat.

No one can claim we know all there is to know about nutrition, obesity and healthy eating as there are still gaps in our knowledge. But what can now be confidently asserted is that the healthiest diet – the one which most reduces the risk of a wide range of diseases – is also the safest and most effective one to return you to your ideal weight and keep you there. This is good news – after all, everyone wants to be slim and healthy, not thin and ill.

It isn't just what you eat and how much you exercise that determines whether or not you're overweight. The other factors are explained in this book. Doctors are often confronted with people who are fat who say, 'But I don't eat enough to keep a sparrow alive' or 'Well, we're all big in our family'. It is true that there are some people who can eat what they like and not put on an ounce and others who put on a pound if they so much as look at a cream cake (not strictly true, but you get my drift!). But comparing yourself with other people isn't at all helpful; if you do belong in the 'eating like a sparrow' category, you certainly have my sympathy but you also have my support.

This book gives you the knowledge you need to take control of your own body and your own life. Don't be fatalistic about being fat; it may be harder for you than for others, but if you want to be slim, and commit yourself to it, then you will succeed.

You need to understand why you're fat and this understanding isn't beyond you. Science and medicine can be understood by everyone – and don't believe white-coated professionals who, in their own interest, pretend otherwise. Being overweight can be explained in one sentence. If you take in more energy (calories) in your food than your body needs for your particular lifestyle, then your body will lay down that surplus energy as fat. The *only* way to lose weight is to take in less energy or to expend more. Please, please don't let anyone tell you any different. So many people want to believe in a magic 'something' which will help them lose weight but it doesn't exist. If you want to believe in something, why not believe in fact rather than in fiction?

- If you cut down the amount of fat you eat, you will take in fewer calories.
- If you cut down the amount of sugar you eat, you will take in fewer calories.
- If you increase the amount of fibre you eat, you will be able to cut down fat and sugar without feeling hungry.
- If you increase your amount of physical activity, you will burn up more calories.

These are the principles on which the BBC Diet is based: if you follow them, you *will* lose weight.

This book explains why those facts are true and how to put those principles into practice in your own life. After you've read it, you'll understand why we get fat and how to get slim. You won't be at the mercy of quacks and charlatans and fad diets. You won't have to carry a diet plan or calorie chart around for ever. You will be in charge of your own body, your own health, your own life.

If you feel fat, your body is trying to tell you something: lose weight. Here's how. . .

HEIGHT-WEIGHT CHART

Find where you are on the chart by taking a line from the left-hand or right-hand side which gives your height. Follow this until it meets your weight line coming from the base or top of the chart. If you are perfect then the two lines meet in the middle of the 'acceptable' area. If you're not quite perfect then work out how far you are from the ideal.

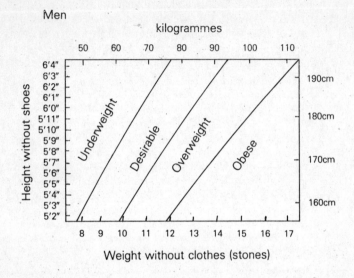

Men

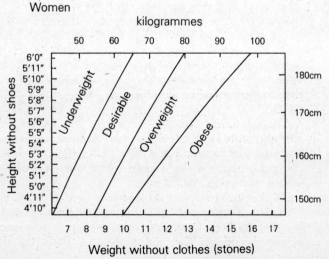

Women

CHAPTER 2

A NATION OF FATTIES

How many people do you know who are trying to lose weight at the moment? Or is an easier question, how many people do you know who are *not* trying to lose weight at the moment? It's been reported by the advertising industry that, at any one time, 65 per cent of British women and 30 per cent of British men are trying to lose weight. A third of the population are regular users of one or more slimming products. It seems that it's the norm in this country to be overweight. There is, as doctors often say when confronted with something they don't fully understand, a lot of it about!

This chapter tells you how to recognise if you're 'officially' overweight and what those 'what you should weigh' charts really mean. It also details the medical risks associated with being fat and considers our attitudes to obesity and body shape.

If you know you're overweight, know you want to lose weight and don't want to know about medical risks, you can jump to the next chapter which tells you why nature or fate has picked you out to be fat and not your thin friends.

THE SCALE OF THE PROBLEM

Obviously most people don't need anyone to tell them whether or not they're overweight: they just know. On the basis of the statistics above, at least two-thirds of women and one third of men 'know' they're overweight and there may be many more who feel that they are overweight but decide to do nothing about it. More ojective evidence confirms the massive scale of the problem: about half of the middle-aged people in this country may be classified as being above their ideal weight.

You can assess if you're overweight and by how much by consulting the Height-Weight Chart opposite. This chart tells you your ideal weight range. The ideal weight for people of a particular height is that weight which is associated with the lowest disease and death rates.

It's helpful to know how these kinds of charts were compiled. They're not based on average weights: in fact, as has already been implied, average weight in this country is above the ideal. The charts are the basis for defining acceptable weights both in this country, and in the USA, and are founded on surveys undertaken earlier this century by an American insurance company which related weight to the risk of death. The original charts were analysed according to the policy holders' subjective assessment of their own frame size, i.e. whether it was small, medium or large (but with no one defining exactly what that meant). Both British and American expert committees have since decided that weights within the whole range given for small, medium and large frame sizes should be considered acceptable: this is why the ideal weight range is so wide, and why the same charts can apply to both men and women. But if you choose the upper limit of the large frame size as the upper limit of ideal this is rather on the generous side. So, if you're pondering whether or not you're really overweight, be hard on yourself!

Obesity is the medical term for being very overweight, i.e. in the fourth range, 'fat', in our chart. Obesity comes from Latin words meaning 'over-eating', so it's a contentious term, as we shall see. Strictly speaking it means a condition of excess body fat, but few definitions are based on measuring or even estimating the fat content of the body. Most studies on obesity have depended on measuring weight compared with height, as does our chart. This is then used as a rather rough and ready assessment of the body's fat content and, of course, also has implications for body shape (see below).

Two further points here

- As already mentioned, the chart is perhaps on the generous side, allowing the upper range of the ideal to be rather high.
- You can aim to get to the bottom of your ideal weight range safely enough but if you feel you want to weigh *less* than the ideal, consult your doctor so you can get a professional opinion on whether or not you're overweight.

BODY SHAPE

Many people, particularly women, may be dissatisfied with the shape of their body and feel that they are fat even though their weight may fall in the ideal range for their height.

There is an unfairness here. When men get fat, they usually become 'apples' with excess weight around their middle – a beer belly is the typical way men get fat. When women get fat, they usually become 'pears' – the extra weight goes on their hips and thighs. 'Apple' fat is usually easier to lose than 'pear' fat as it is mainly laid down in response to overeating, whereas 'pear' fat is also controlled by female sex hormones. Women, of course, can get 'apple' fat as well. The familiar problem of the last few pounds of weight being just where you don't want it does apply more to women than to men, as their shape is partly due to their sex hormones.

You may have to accept the fact, even when you're down to your ideal weight and have toned your muscles up by regular exercise, that you still may not be happy with the shape of your body. Don't compare yourself with others; slim bodies do vary in shape. Some people go in at the waist and others don't; some have big thighs and others have small ones. This is nothing to do with fat and excess weight, but everything to do with individual variation. It is rather like not liking the shape or size of your nose: losing weight won't affect it!

We all have 'imperfections' so seeking for perfection is fruitless. When you've lost weight don't dwell on the bits of your body you're still not happy with – concentrate on and emphasise the bits you like!

THE MEDICAL RISKS OF OBESITY

There is no doubt that, over a period of years, being overweight will have an effect on your health and make a number of diseases more likely. These risks become serious for those who come under the medical definition of obese, that is those who are more than 20 per cent above their ideal weight, but some of the effects increase progressively when you are just slightly above your ideal weight.

Overweight and raised blood cholesterol

Being overweight pushes up the level of fats, including cholesterol, in the blood. This then increases the chance of a heart attack or a stroke: when you lose weight, your blood cholesterol level falls.

Overweight and heart disease

Being overweight also increases your risk of heart disease in several other ways. Everyone in this country is more likely to die of a heart attack than anything else and the more overweight you are, the more your risk of heart disease increases. For men aged 35-44 years, it has been shown that a 10 per cent increase in weight increases the chance of heart disease by 38 per cent. A 20 per cent increase in weight pushes up the risk of a heart attack by 86 per cent. Women are not immune from this effect, although in this age group their risk of heart disease is less than men's. This protective effect is thought to be caused by female sex hormones. The difference does disappear after the menopause.

Overweight and high blood pressure

Being even slightly overweight can cause a rise in blood pressure and for some susceptible people it will be quite a serious rise. High blood pressure increases the chance of heart attacks and strokes but losing weight often has the beneficial effect of returning blood pressure to normal. Indeed, doctors often advise patients with high blood pressure to try to lose some weight as their blood pressure may then return to normal without the need to take any medication.

Overweight and diabetes

There are two types of diabetes: one which can occur in young people and needs injections of insulin to treat it and another which begins in middle or old age and can be treated by tablets or diet or both. This latter type is caused by being overweight, and the risk of developing diabetes increases with the degree of obesity.

Overweight and gall-stones

The fatter you are, the more likely you are to develop stones in your gall bladder. This is due to the greater amount of cholesterol that fat people tend to have: the cholesterol is precipitated out of the bile to form stones.

Another factor which makes gall-stones more likely in fat people is the use of inappropriate and outdated slimming diets such as low carbohydrate or low-fibre diets which tend to encourage the formation of gall-stones.

Overweight and cancer

Statistically there are greater risks of developing certain types of cancer in those who are overweight. In men, there's a greater chance of developing cancer of the colon, the rectum and the prostate. In women, the likelihood of developing cancer of the breast, womb and cervix is increased. All of these are quite common cancers and there's also an increased risk of developing some less common ones such as cancer of the gall bladder.

Overweight and lung disease

One of the commonest complaints of those who are overweight is breathlessness on mild exertion, such as walking uphill or upstairs. Various measurements of the lungs' ability to function properly show that their capacity deteriorates as obesity develops. If you're overweight, you're more likely to develop a chest infection after having an operation.

Overweight and arthritis

The most common form of arthritis is osteoarthritis which tends to affect everyone as they get older as it's a mechanical effect of the joints wearing out. This form of arthritis improves after losing weight.

Gout is a rarer form of arthritis, the risk of which increases in men who are very overweight.

Overweight and varicose veins

In those who are obese, or severely overweight (that is, 20 per cent above their ideal weight), the risk of developing varicose veins doubles.

Overweight and irregular periods

Being overweight can lead to various menstrual abnormalities and being severely overweight can cause heavy and painful periods. The hormonal imbalance that is caused by being overweight can also lead to the distressing symptom of hirsutism: an increase and change in the normal distribution of body hair.

Overweight and feeling tired and weary

Feeling tired may not sound as serious as some of the other complications of being overweight, but it can be quite debilitating and seriously diminish the quality of life. It's not a surprising symptom: if you're a couple of stone overweight, it's as if you're carrying around a couple of heavy suitcases all the time. This excess weight will also probably give you backache and make a slipped disc more likely.

Overweight and mental health

Being fat isn't just a matter of illness and getting slim isn't just a matter of physical health. For some people, being fat and wanting to be slim is the most important thing in their life. Being fat can make them so unhappy that they start overeating for comfort which, like a vicious spiral, just makes them fatter still.

If being fat is getting you depressed or if you know you're indulging in huge binges, you need professional help. It's important for you to see your G.P.

LOSING WEIGHT AND IMPROVING YOUR HEALTH

Whatever your reasons for wanting to lose weight – and they may be very important – one compelling reason, as you've seen, is that you will improve your health and decrease the risks of developing a wide range of diseases.

CHAPTER 3

WHY AM I FAT?

How is it that you, who desperately nibble at lettuce leaves and low-fat cottage cheese, are fat while your friend, who gorges on chips, chocolate and cream cakes, is thin? It's unfair, yes: life is unfair in this as in so many other ways. This chapter explains why some of us are fat and some are thin – not only individuals but whole nations. Once you understand why your body is the way it is, you've got the knowledge and therefore the power to do something about it. You can't change the person you are, but I'll be explaining why you need only be a product of your genes, and not a prisoner of them.

WHY WE'VE BEEN GETTING FATTER

For more than forty years now – since the end of the Second World War – there's been a progressive increase in the average weight for height of adults in the United Kingdom. Unfortunately this hasn't been due to an increase in healthy muscle: over that time the average amount of body fat in adults has gone up by 10 per cent. Remember that's an average: it is not evenly spread and those millions of pounds of excess fat are found on the *half* of the population which is overweight.

Looking at what happens to whole populations over decades is very useful for understanding health and disease. One of the biggest puzzles in medical science is why some people get infections or diseases and others don't. Before vaccinations rendered the disease so rare, not everyone exposed to the polio virus developed polio. In the middle ages, the Bubonic Plague, known as the Black Death, wiped out at least a quarter of the population of Europe but it didn't kill everyone. Why? We're here to tell the tale and ask the question.

The best modern example of a killer disease is the epidemic of our own century: heart disease. This was very rare until 50 or 60 years ago and its prevalence now can only be explained by understanding that the whole population has changed its behaviour by, for example, smoking more, exercising less and eating more fat. That doesn't mean that *everyone* will get a heart attack, but it does mean that where the behaviour which increases the risk of heart disease is common, then very many people in the population will develop it. They are the people who are 'susceptible'; the majority, it seems, in the case of heart disease. The same thing is seen if we look at the incidence of high blood pressure: most people eat a high salt diet in this country and for some that can help to cause high blood pressure. Others can eat a lot of salt without any effect on their blood pressure. Therefore if the *average* level of salt eaten in the country came down, then the number of people suffering from high blood pressure – the 'incidence' of the disease – would also be reduced.

This is a difficult concept but an extremely important one. If the whole population changed its lifestyle in certain key respects, heart disease would no longer be a mass killer. But if everyone had reduced their risk of a heart attack to the absolute minimum, a *small* number of people would still get heart disease, and they are fated to get it no matter what they do. *Most* of us, though, are in charge of our own destiny in this respect.

The same applies to the problem of being overweight. In our present society it's a mass problem affecting about half of the population and, perhaps even two-thirds or more of us are susceptible to some degree of weight gain.

But although this is true throughout the affluent West, it is not the case for all populations. The vast majority of people in India or China live a rural, peasant lifestyle and their diet consists largely of rice, pulses and vegetables with very little meat. Most of them are involved in manual labour and very, very few of them are overweight. Of course there are *some* people in those countries who are: either those who are following a more westernised lifestyle and diet or those who belong to the 'irreducible minimum'. In the case of being overweight, these are people who have glandular or metabolic illnesses which account for their obesity.

These illnesses are very rare: they account for 5 per cent or less of the people in the United Kingdom who are very overweight (20 per cent or more over their ideal weight.) So for the majority of us who are overweight it's our lifestyle which has 'brought out' this hidden susceptibility to fatness.

Fat babies become fat adults

There is some evidence that the way we are fed in infancy and childhood may have long-term effects. In fact, it has been suggested that the increase in weight of young adults in the 1980s reflects inappropriate infant feeding in the 1950s and 1960s. It has been demonstrated that bottle-fed babies are particularly likely to show an excessive weight gain. Of course, with babies, unlike adults, big is beautiful; babies are never fat, only 'bonny'. Babies who are fat are more likely to turn into children who are fat who, in turn, are more likely to grow into adults who are fat. It's not inevitable that all fat babies and children will grow into fat adults, but it's more likely. So we need to keep an eye on our children's weight as well as our own.

About seven per cent of pre-teenage children are overweight and the problem gets greater as children get older. Half of British 20-year-olds are already at the upper limit of their ideal weight or going over it. By the age of 25, 31 per cent of men and 27 per cent of women are substantially overweight – that is, more than 10 per cent above their ideal weight and so at risk of ill-health.

Why you are fat

Are we programmed to be fat, then? Should we be fatalistic and decide to be fat but happy? In fact, like so many other characteristics – our height, our intelligence, our personality – being overweight or slim is determined by a combination of the characteristics which we inherit from our parents and the circumstances in which we live. Some of us (very few) are programmed to be fat; some of us, (in fact, most of us) are programmed to be fat or thin depending on the sort of life we live; and the lucky others are programmed to be thin no matter what they do.

There are four key things which determine whether the majority of us are fat or thin. Two of them are largely under our own control and it seems that we can influence the third to a small but significant degree as well.

The two under our control are
- appetite and the amount and type of food we eat
- the amount of physical activity we undertake.

The one we may be able to influence is
- our basal metabolic rate (BMR) or 'tickover' speed.

And the other key factor, which we do not know how far we can influence, is

- thermogenesis or the ability of the body to burn up excess calories as heat.

APPETITE AND THE AMOUNT OF FOOD WE EAT

Modern planes can fly for thousands of miles on automatic pilot and can even, using computer-controlled autoland, put down perfectly on a runway. Alternatively, the controls can be under the control of the pilot's thinking human mind.

This is a useful analogy for many of our body's functions: automatic pilot or control by the unconscious mind at one extreme and manual control or control by the conscious, thinking mind at the other. In fact, most functions are a combination of the two. For example, our heart rate is almost wholly controlled by the unconscious mind: we can't think 'go faster' and make it do so (though, in fact, certain relaxation techniques can reduce it). Then there's breathing: we never need to think about it and it happens automatically every few seconds for as long as we live, but we can override the automatic pilot whenever we wish by deciding to take a deep breath. If we try to override by holding our breath, the automatic pilot switches on again. The automatic pilot is programmed to adjust if we need more air in our lungs: when we start running, we breathe more often and more deeply.

Similarly, there's an interplay between the automatic and manual control, between the unconscious and conscious, in the control of our appetite, the amount of food we eat and also its type. But unlike our heart rate and breathing, the automatic, unconscious control of our appetite seems neither very important nor very precise. More important seems to be what we like, what's available, and the social and family pressures on us to eat particular amounts and types of food.

Even so, some unconscious control certainly does exist although not a great deal is known about it. There appears to be an appetite control centre in the hypothalamus of the brain which is influenced by hormones produced in the stomach and intestines in response to food. This is additional to the feeling of fullness we experience when food goes into the stomach and fills and distends it. In the early stages of man's evolution, the control centres may have been important not in telling them to eat less food but in telling them to eat more.

Before the days of well-stacked larders, supermarket shelves and fast-food counters, our cave-people ancestors didn't know where their next meal was coming from. The appetite control centre was important in urging them to find not only the right amount of food but also enough of the right *kinds* of food.

Feeding experiments with young babies have shown that this primitive control still exists. Pre-weighed feeding bottles of milk were delivered to the homes of these babies. The mothers were asked to feed the babies until they stopped of their own accord and not to coax them to finish their bottles. Over a period of time, unknown to the mothers, the milk delivered to some of the babies was diluted so that it contained fewer calories per fluid ounce. The babies fed on the diluted milk rapidly increased their intake so that their energy intake remained the same as that of the babies who were receiving smaller amounts of more concentrated milk.

Even babies don't all behave in the same way: fat babies respond favourably to being given feeds with increasing concentrations of glucose, whereas thin babies tend to shun sweet solutions. It also seems that the relationship between the mother and the baby is important; babies can learn food habits so that they come to like sweet things and eat more than they would if no parental coaxing took place.

Even though our eating habits can be affected by many other factors, it seems that the appetite control centre does have some restraining influence over the amount we eat – provided that we are eating in a 'natural' way. In the next chapter, we'll see how much of our food is 'unnatural' because it is refined and therefore many more calories can be packed in during our meals than either our unconscious appetite control centre or our conscious minds realise. That chapter explains the paradox of how we can feel full and satisfied after two different meals containing very different amounts of calories.

Some people, as we know, can stuff in calories with impunity. Even if they eat far more calories than their body needs, they can compensate and put on hardly any extra weight. For example, some lean men usually consuming about 3000 calories a day can be fed food containing 6-8000 calories a day for several weeks and increase their weight by only ten per cent. If they then continue to consume 5000 calories a day, they neither gain nor lose weight; in other words they have adapted to the new circumstances and once again they are in energy balance. A body in energy balance neither gains nor loses weight because the number of calories coming in as food energy is the same as the number of calories being used for bodily functions and activity.

Alas, most of us aren't as fortunate as this. If we were to start packing in excess calories it would be quite some time before our body adapted and, if we were eventually to get back into energy balance, we would be 2 to 3 stone (15 to 20 kg) or more above our ideal weight.

Important though it is, the amount and type of food we eat is not the sole determining factor in the weight we put on.

PHYSICAL ACTIVITY

The striking difference between us and our forebears in the last and every preceding generation is that we are far less physically active. Our grandparents couldn't so much accuse us of the deadly sin of gluttony but rather of sloth. In our push-button, mechanised world we can get away with hardly moving our bodies at all if we don't want to. Even those of us who do manual work have far more machines to help us than the last generation. The rest of us expend very few calories in our day-to-day work and in our leisure time the only exercise we may get is flicking a finger at the remote control which changes channels on our television set!

It may be that you feel that you're no more inactive than your thin friends (though there is evidence that those who are overweight tend to be less active), but unfortunately that's not the point and it's not a useful comparison to make. The population as a whole is far less active than that of a generation ago and so again those who don't gain weight are the lucky ones whose bodies have adapted to the new conditions.

OUR METABOLIC RATE

Not only does the amount of energy or calories we take in as food and the amount of energy we expend in physical activity differ from person to person, the amount of energy needed by the body simply to keep itself alive varies greatly too, so that some people may use up twice the amount of energy used by others of equivalent size. This energy is used up in the internal processes of the body such as breathing, digesting and keeping the body temperature normal. It's the energy used before we even lift a finger and is needed for the body-machine to 'tick-over' or 'idle'. The degree of this tick-over speed, which varies from person to person, is called the basal or resting metabolic rate (BMR).

It used to be thought that people leading a normal life expended energy at the rate of at least 1.5 times their BMR. But recent research has shown that young healthy women expend energy at an average of only 1.38 times their BMR – that is the total amount of energy they used up was only 38 per cent greater than if they had stayed in bed all day. This, of course, is further proof of our increasingly inactive lifestyle; this trend, which has been evident for some time, is in fact even more marked than was first thought. As our food intake tends to be higher than is needed for the amount of activity we do, those with a low BMR are most at risk of gaining excess weight and becoming fat.

Showing that people who are already overweight have a low BMR is more difficult, as the BMR itself is dependent on body weight. Lean tissue has a higher metabolic rate than fat tissue, but people who are overweight, because they are bigger overall, tend to have more lean tissue as well as more fat tissue than their lean counterparts.

But how our own BMR compares with other people's isn't really helpful. There are, as we're seeing, many variables which determine whether we're fat or thin and the ways they interact and balance with each other in each individual are not yet fully understood. The vital thing – which *is* absolutely clear – is that our BMR is not static, it's not 'set' at some point which is unchangeable.

There are two very important points about the BMR which those who want to lose weight need to know:

● Our BMR changes when we go on a diet which has fewer calories, less energy, than our normal diet. In response to fewer calories the body *lowers* its BMR because it starts to think not 'I'm losing weight' but 'hard times are coming; food seems to be less plentiful; where is my next meal coming from; I'd better start conserving energy.' This phenomenon, which is discussed in Chapter Five, is crucial to an understanding of losing weight effectively and explains those things the seasoned dieter dreads after the first few, easy, pounds have been shed: the 'plateau' effect (i.e. increasing difficulty in losing weight while remaining on what seems a semi-starvation diet) and the startling rebound effect of weight gain when a diet ends.

• Our BMR *increases* in response to increased physical activity. Not only do we burn off excess calories doing our exercise, but the increased BMR continues even after we have stopped exercise. Again, this is discussed in Chapter Eight on exercise. This effect lasts for several hours, and there's even evidence that when sustained and vigorous exercise is regular, the increased BMR continues on a more or less permanent basis. Of course, the amount of the increase varies from person to person, but even a modest increase should at least counteract the body's tendency to decrease the BMR when we start cutting calories.

This is the key to the success of the BBC Diet and why it is superior to all those diets which just cut calories. By combining exercise with cutting down the fatty and sugary foods which pile on the calories, you'll not only slim more quickly and more effectively but your weight loss is also more likely to be permanent. Above all, you'll feel fitter and be healthier.

THERMOGENESIS

This is the body's ability to burn up excess calories taken in as food energy and produce heat. It's been postulated that one of the differences between thin and fat people is their efficiency in carrying out thermogenesis, so that, while thin people are able to burn up their excess calories, fat people are not able to do so and instead store them as fat.

There are weak links to this argument. Most of the experimental work has been done on rats; and thermogenesis is much more important in controlling the body temperature of small animals like rats than it is in large animals like man.

Thermogenesis is thought to take place where reserves of one particular type of fat – 'brown fat' – have been laid down. You may have heard about 'brown fat' or 'brown adipose tissue' (BAT) when it was a fashionable discussion point a few years ago. At one time it was paraded as the miracle key to unlock the problem of overweight for ever: it isn't.

There is evidence that BAT is important in rats, but not,

unfortunately, in humans. Brown fat is found only at certain sites in the body and overall it accounts for only a tiny percentage of our body fat.

More research needs to be done and, indeed, is being done, on this whole subject in relation to human beings but two things which are now emerging give even more encouragement for the way of losing weight advocated by the BBC Diet:

- Thermogenesis seems to occur partly in response to eating food and its rate may depend on the *type* of food eaten. There's some evidence now that calories may be burned up more slowly on a high-fat diet. Experiments with animals seem to indicate that high-fat diets encourage weight gain. By following the low-fat BBC Diet you'll not only be reducing the number of calories you eat, but may also be burning up those calories you do eat more efficiently.
- Experimental evidence shows that diet-induced thermogenesis may be increased by taking exercise. This is in addition to both the higher BMR induced by exercise and to the calories the exercise itself burns off. With this two-pronged attack, the BBC Diet gives you the very best way to lose those excess pounds.

CHAPTER 4

FOOD, GLORIOUS FOOD

Food is one of the great pleasures of my life — is it of yours? Or do you regard food as the enemy? Are you engaged in trench warfare against it?

Food should be enjoyable: regarding it as a great temptation which must be firmly resisted while you're dieting is totally counter-productive. You're only going to succumb on a grand scale when you stop.

What is more guilt-provoking to a failed dieter than eating a big fat cake oozing with whipped cream? But having negative feelings towards food is destructive and doesn't help to shed one ounce. Our attitude towards food should be positive but realistic and knowledgeable. We can be friends with all foods, but some foods should be our bosom buddies while others should only be 'sometimes' friends. Once you begin to approach eating with this attitude, you're in control of the food you eat — it's not in control of you.

To be in control of our eating we need to understand food and the effect different sorts of food have, not only on our weight and body shape, but also on our health. One of the keys to successful slimming is knowing that it's not only the *amount* of food we eat that is important, but also the *type* of food.

This is the good news about the BBC Diet: we can still enjoy eating while following it and not suffer from hunger pangs. We'll not only be losing weight but, as we change to a healthier diet, we'll become fitter and more healthy as well.

This chapter tells you all you need to know about calories, fat, sugar, carbohydrates, protein and fibre. It'll explain the principles on which the BBC Diet is based and why those principles make this not only the most effective and easiest diet to follow, but also the healthiest.

CALORIES

The seasoned dieter knows that calories are the enemy's front-line troops. It's strange that 'calories' have such a negative image whereas 'energy' has such a positive one. The food manufacturer who comes up with a 'low-calorie' and 'high-energy' food is going to make a fortune. In fact, it's impossible because 'calorie' and 'energy' in this context are exactly the same thing: calories are the units in which we measure the energy which is present in the food we eat. Remember that next time you see an advert for a drink or chocolate bar proudly proclaiming 'high in energy' and think how its sales would fall if the equally truthful statement 'high in calories' were proclaimed instead.

The scientific definition of the calorie is that it is the amount of energy required to increase the temperature of 1 gram of water by 1 degree centigrade. The 'calorie' that we normally talk about, and we refer to throughout this book, is really a kilocalorie, because it would raise the temperature of 1 kilogram (nearly two pints) of water by 1 degree centigrade. So 100 calories of the sort we normally talk about (which are really kilocalories) is the energy which would bring to the boil two pints of water – that's quite a lot of energy!

We really need only concern ourselves with calories in their hundreds. It's not going to make a great deal of difference to your weight loss if you're consuming 1100 rather than 1000 calories (and there's at least this variation in natural food anyway). Certainly to fret about single calories is crazy: four peas, two baked beans, two slices of cucumber all contain about one calorie; $\frac{1}{2}$ oz (15 g) of butter, on the other hand, contains 100 calories! This shows that it is important to recognise those kinds of foods which are dense in calories and those that are not.

The BBC Diet, unlike many others, doesn't tell you to count calories. There are very good reasons for this.

- you don't need to count calories, you just need to consume fewer of them. By following the principles of the BBC Diet, you'll do this automatically.
- it's been shown many times – and perhaps you know it's true –that people with normal busy lives can't keep an accurate record of the number of calories they eat. Even if they're told to weigh everything, there are always some things that slip in unweighed and 'estimated'. Even when doctors and nutritionists try to do this, their estimates are often way out. Calorie counting is also boring and quite time-consuming as I found out during the week I did it while following the principles of the BBC Diet.
- It's far more important to understand the basic principles so that you can then apply them to any situation you find

yourself in. Then you're in control of the situation and not blindly following a set of calorie-counting rules.

But although you don't need to count calories, you do need to have a 'calorie awareness'. You do need to know the types of foods which can knock you for six with their punch of calories and those types of food you really have to stuff yourself with in order to take in calories in triple or even double figures. There's more about these types of food later in the chapter but first here are the few simple facts about calories that you need to know:

- all food contains some calories. Don't allow yourself to be fooled into thinking that some foods don't have any calories. Fat, protein and carbohydrates all contain calories.
- all drinks (except water) contain calories. This may be an insignificant number, as in black tea or coffee and low-cal drinks which are largely water, flavouring and artificial sweetener, or quite a significant number as in alcoholic drinks which can dramatically increase your daily calorie intake without your being aware of it.
- although all foods contain some calories, some contain many more than others or are 'calorie-dense'. For example, ten pounds (4.5 kg) of apples have fewer calories than one pound (450 kg) of chocolates. This is good news for slimmers because if you choose your foods carefully (and the BBC Diet tells you how) you can eat your fill, not feel hungry and reduce your calorie intake – all at the same time.
- fat and sugar are the two biggest 'calorie-packers' – they deliver a large dose of calories in a small space and a small weight of food. For example, two teaspoonsful of sugar contain as many calories as 4 oz (100 g) of peas, while 1 oz (25 g) of butter contains more calories than 10 oz (275 g) of potatoes.
- fibre is a great 'calorie-saver'. It bulks out food and causes it to be less dense in calories weight-for-weight. It's fibre that causes those peas, for example, to be so much less calorie-dense than sugar.

You can now see why the BBC Diet is based on three simple principles
- cutting down fat
- cutting down sugar
- increasing fibre

If you do this – and the later chapters tell you how – you will automatically reduce your calorie intake and you can't fail to lose weight.

All diets that work depend on cutting calories – there's no way round this; there's no magic pill that can melt fat away. The BBC Diet combines cutting calories with exercise which increases the rate at which excess calories are burnt off – thereby making the diet even more effective. Chapter Five looks at other diets and methods of losing weight and explains how even those diets which proclaim you can eat anything you want and lose weight have in-built tricks which decrease your calorie intake. If they didn't, they wouldn't work. Although other diets may be as effective as the BBC Diet in losing weight, the BBC Diet is the healthiest diet you can follow and is designed not only to help you to lose that weight but also to keep it off.

WHY THE AVERAGE BRITISH DIET MAKES US FAT

As we've already seen, our problem is that our lifestyles are becoming so inactive that we're consuming excessive calories for our way of life.

When we consider our health, it's not only the number of calories that is important, though, but also where these calories are coming from. Since the beginning of this century, our diet has changed so that we now eat more fat and less 'complex' carbohydrates – like the starches and fibre found in fruit, vegetables and cereals – and we're now eating vastly more sugar. The amount of protein we eat has remained about the same.

Some of these changes have happened because we have more money to spend on food and some foods have become relatively much cheaper. Fashion, and different views of what's healthy, have also played their part in altering the pattern of the food we eat. But some of the most important changes have happened because of the way much of the food is now sold to us. We're now eating a lot of food which may not have been touched by human hand but has certainly been touched by a great deal of machinery – processed food.

Processing food – refining it, taking things out of it, putting other things into it, mixing it together and packaging it – has often meant making it cheaper. Sometimes it's made it more nutritious too, though not always.

For example, when the machine milling of rice was introduced in the Far East, it was considered a great advance and people found the resulting polished rice, with the husk taken off, much more palatable. But an important vitamin, B_1 or thiamine, is present in significant amounts in the outer husk and for people living on a rice-based diet this is an important source of the vitamin. By eating the polished rice, now lacking in B_1, they began to get the disease beri-beri.

This story illustrates how our bodies may sometimes be tricked. Polished rice tasted as good as whole rice and there was nothing to show that it was lacking something – until people became ill.

This is one of the problems with processed foods: they may be lacking some of the nutrients that whole, unrefined, 'natural' foods supply. (Though it should be said that some processed foods have nutrients added to them; for example, vitamins are added by law to margarine.) There's another aspect to processed foods of particular concern to those who want to lose weight.

The problem is the opposite of a lack of nutrients – it's a surfeit of calories. Processing food can cause large numbers of calories to be packed into a small space, because it so often includes those two 'calorie-packers': fat and sugar. Take the case of the ten pounds of apples having fewer calories than one pound of chocolates. It's fairly easy – isn't it? – to eat a pound of chocolates at one sitting but it's almost impossible to eat ten pounds of apples. Whole, natural, unrefined food like an apple has a low calorie to weight ratio, or low energy-density, because it's packed with fibre and water. It's impossible to take in too many calories by eating this type of food, because before we have done so, we feel full and satisfied. But refined foods often have a very high calorie to weight ratio, or high energy-density, and so we can, weight for weight, eat far more and therefore take in a large number of calories before we feel full.

As already noted, fat and sugar are the two culprits in making processed food energy-dense and, like the terrible twins, they often make an appearance together. Chocolate, for example, is largely sweetened fat. A large quantity of the products of the food industry rely on sweetening fat, as in chocolate biscuits and cakes, or on salting it, as in crisps, sausages, pies and pasties, in order to make it palatable. If we were eating unprocessed food that we could recognise we wouldn't possibly eat so much fat. A meat pie or sausage may deliver half or more of its large dose of calories in fat. Fat is cheaper than meat, so it's mixed with meat and other things in order to become palatable and to make us buy it.

There's another twist to this story, which is important for everyone's health whether or not they need to lose weight. We don't rely on our food just for calories or energy but also for nutrients, for minerals, for vitamins, for essential amino acids – all substances that our body can't manufacture. As our food has become high in energy-density, it's also become low in nutrient-density. This is going to be an increasing danger in the future. If our intake of calories falls, as our physical activity reduces, we may be in danger of not getting enough nutrients from the food we eat. Calorie for calorie we get less nutrients from processed food with high energy-density than we do from natural wholefood with low energy-density. By 'natural whole food', I don't mean food from health shops; you can buy natural whole food in any supermarket. It's food you can recognise immediately and see what plant or tree it grew on or what fish or animal it came from.

So, although we may be taking in enough calories – or too many – we may still be malnourished if our food isn't sufficiently rich with the nutrients we need.

This is the danger of some diets which cut down the calories but also cut down valuable nutrients. However, the balanced and healthy BBC Diet avoids this and even though you're cutting down the calories, you should be increasing the nutrients by following our guidelines.

FAT

I remember reading a book on dieting when I was a medical student which proclaimed 'Fat doesn't create fat; in fact, fat burns up fat.' One thing I did learn as a medical student is that medical knowledge rarely flies in the face of common sense. Fat is loaded with calories and is the number one culprit in making us fat – and don't let anyone tell you otherwise. On average, each of us in Britain gets 40 per cent of our calories from fat – 40 per cent! Not only is this extremely bad for our figures, it's also bad for our health.

Fat and health

The British people's high intake of fat is now linked to the mass epidemic of heart disease. In particular, our consumption of saturated fat causes a high level of cholesterol in the blood which, in turn, helps to clog up our arteries and form the basis for a heart attack or stroke. Saturated fat is predominant in fats of animal origin such as meat, butter, cream, cheese and milk. It has a different chemical structure from polyunsaturated fats which predominate in fats from vegetable and fish origin such as sunflower oil and the fat in herrings and mackerel.

As far as losing weight is concerned, fat *is* fat and we need to cut down our intake to reduce the calories. It's sensible though to follow the health guidelines and cut down proportionately more on saturated fat, replacing it with a lesser quantity of polyunsaturates – for example, by using an oil high in polyunsaturates like sunflower oil. On health grounds alone, we should *all* follow the official medical recommendations to cut down our fat consumption by at least a quarter (this is the official target for the next decade); and while we're dieting we need to cut down even further. It would be undesirable – and in fact next to impossible – to cut fat from our diet completely. There are certain types of fat which are essential in small quantities and some vitamins are present in fat because they are fat- and not water-soluble.

Hidden fat to all-too visible fat

You may be surprised, even disbelieving, that 40 per cent of our calories come from fat. How can that be, if you perhaps don't even like fat? We all consume far more fat than we think and much of it is 'hidden'. It's not just the fat we can see that counts, but also all that that we can't see – chocolate is one-third fat, so is cheddar cheese; roast shoulder of lamb is a quarter fat and even 'lean' grilled rump steak is 12 per cent fat. Also, fat contains twice as many calories, weight for weight, as carbohydrate and protein.

To get slim, you just need to develop your fat detector – later in the book the BBC Diet guidelines tell you exactly how to reduce your fat intake – but meanwhile here is where the fat in the average British diet comes from:

- 27 per cent from meat and meat products
- 25 per cent from butter and margarine

- 13 per cent from milk
- 13 per cent from cooking oils and fats
- 6 per cent from biscuits, cakes and pastries
- 5 per cent from cheese and cream
- 11 per cent from other foods

PROTEIN

Protein is an essential part of our diet, but it's virtually impossible for someone in the United Kingdom to go short of it – in fact we eat about twice as much protein as we need. The proportion of protein in our diet has remained about the same over this century, and the consensus of medical opinion is that we should keep the consumption at about the present level. With present-day medical knowledge, the high-protein diets recommended in the past make no nutritional sense. Weight for weight, protein contains more calories than carbohydrate.

The problem for those wanting to lose weight is that protein is very often bound up with fat. As we've just seen, the protein in roast shoulder of lamb is bound up with 26 per cent fat and the protein in Cheddar cheese is bound up with 33 per cent fat. So what the dieter needs to do is find good sources of protein which aren't bound up with fat. Obviously some lean meat is all right, but chicken and white fish are even better – high in protein but low in fat. It's a myth, by the way, that only meat provides 'first class' protein – the protein of chicken and fish are just as nutritious. And by pairing beans, peas or lentils with rice or wholemeal bread or pasta, you end up with a complete protein meal – as well as providing only the tiniest traces of fat.

SUGAR

'Pure, white and deadly' as one famous professor of nutrition has labelled it.

Can you believe you eat over 100 lb (50 kg) of sugar a year? On average we eat nearly 2 lb (1 kg) of sugar each every week in this country – as much as each person in the last century ate in a whole year. That's about 3500 calories a week – for nothing. We could cut it out of our diet tomorrow and we wouldn't be any the less well-nourished.

Sugar is very calorie- or energy-dense. And those calories

are 'empty': they provide us with virtually no other nutrients at all. The sugar industry tells us sugar provides us with energy; that's true but the other way of saying it is that it provides us with calories and plenty of them. It's a myth that we need sugar for energy: our body can convert any food into energy and calories are just a measure of that energy. We don't need any 'instant' energy from sugar either; our bodies have already thought of that and we have glucose in our bloodstream and glycogen (glucose and water) stored in our liver and muscles instantly available whenever we need them. We'd be dead if we didn't!

It's also a myth that brown sugar is better for you than white; it's not – sugar is sugar. Molasses, glucose, dextrose, syrup, sucrose and fructose and maltose all amount to the same thing – sugar. Sugar is the ideal food for slimmers to cut out completely – it cuts down calories drastically without cutting down on nutrients.

Sugar as we use it is an unnatural product; in nature it comes bound up with fibre – as in fresh fruit for example. As fibre is bulky and filling, it's impossible to consume large quantities of sugar when it comes bound up with fibre. In the manufacturing process, sugar is refined and concentrated, and we can then eat large quantities of it before we feel full.

Half of the sugar the average person eats is out of a packet and we ourselves add it to food; the other half is in manufactured foods. Obviously sugar is added to things like fizzy drinks – ten teaspoonsful or so in an average can – and sweet confectionery but it's also added to breakfast cereals, sauces, chutneys and tinned soups and vegetables. If you start reading food labels you'll be surprised where sugar is shown as an added ingredient.

Do yourself a favour: develop your 'sugar detector'!

One last myth: honey is mostly sugar and water and contains few other nutrients – the most 'magic' ingredient it contains is a large dose of calories. Honey is a refined food too, by the way, but it is refined by bees and not by machines.

VITAMINS AND ESSENTIAL TRACE ELEMENTS

Vitamins and minerals are essential for the healthy functioning of the body, but they are required only in very small doses. It's extremely rare for vitamin deficiencies to occur in western countries like Britain. It can happen if people go on fad diets and eat large quantities of one particular type of food to the exclusion of others. It won't happen to you on the BBC Diet because it is balanced; all the foods we need to eat are there in healthy proportions and so all the vitamins and minerals we need will be present as well.

Minor degrees of iron deficiency may be more common than any vitamin deficiency; this problem occurs mainly in women of childbearing age because of their losses of iron during menstruation. But even here, a balanced diet should provide enough iron for the body's needs.

One thing that is particularly important is to ensure that you're eating plenty of fresh fruit and vegetables and so having an adequate intake of vitamin C. Vitamin C allows the body to absorb the iron that it needs more easily from the food we eat. If our vitamin C intake is adequate – which it will be when following this diet – sufficient iron will be provided by eating some meat and also eating cereals, pulses and vegetables.

The other mineral we need to ensure we get enough of is calcium, essential for the continued growth and health of tissues and bones. We get calcium from a range of foods but simply by drinking ½ pint (300 ml) of skimmed milk a day we are guaranteeing that we are getting all the calcium we need. Even this isn't essential if your intake of food is varied. Skimmed milk contains all the calcium that whole milk does but only a tiny fraction of the fat.

If you're eating a normal and balanced diet you shouldn't have to take expensive vitamin pills or mineral supplements. Your body can use only a certain, small, amount of these elements – and any extra doesn't make you any fitter but just goes to waste. Why not spend the money instead on a nice treat for yourself once you've started losing weight – a non-fattening treat of course!

CARBOHYDRATES AND FIBRE

Seeing these two words linked together may create something of a conflict in your mind, 'Fibre – that's good, isn't it, we should be eating more of it, it helps us to lose weight' and, an echo from the past, 'Carbohydrate, that's bad, lots of carbohydrate means putting on weight'.

If so, it may surprise you to hear that fibre *is* carbohydrate, the unavailable part that we don't digest; what we call carbohydrate is the available part that we do. They always come wrapped up together except in one notorious case – refined sugar. As we've seen, nature meant us to take our carbohydrate gift-wrapped!

This is another source of confusion. Sugar is carbohydrate, but it's a 'simple' one. The other sorts of carbohydrate – the ones we should be eating more of, both for the sake of our health and for losing weight – are 'complex' ones: these are the starches and fibre bound up together in fruit, vegetables, cereals, pulses. Bread – or rather flour – and potatoes are the two basic sources of these complex carbohydrates for us in Britain.

Many of yesterday's diets were low in carbohydrates and lumped refined carbohydrates, notably sugar, in the same category as complex carbohydrates. This was a mistake, as nutritionists and doctors now recognise. Of course, low-carbohydrate diets, if they were successful in cutting calories, did help you to lose weight; but they were an unhealthy way of losing weight and also ineffective in maintaining long-term weight loss.

To people brought up on those old ways of thinking, it's difficult to believe that bread and potatoes are not only allowed on a modern, healthy weight-reducing diet like the BBC's but even encouraged. There is a very sound reason for this: they are filling foods without being fattening. They are not calorie-dense or energy-dense because, weight for weight, they contain far, far fewer calories than fat or sugar. Instead of fattening calories, they contain bulky carbohydrates, starches and fibres which satisfy our hunger. This means that we can't eat too much of them, and so consume too many calories, before we get full.

They do become fattening, though, if we start adding fat to them; when we fry the potatoes as chips, and slap butter on the bread, we start bumping up the calories enormously. But if we don't add fat (or sugar) to them, they are our allies in the fight against the flab.

Fibre – the magic cure?

There's certainly nothing magic about fibre – it isn't like taking a pill which is going to protect us from putting on weight. Increasing fibre is only one part of the BBC Diet; the others – cutting fat and sugar and increasing exercise – are at least as important, if not more so. In some of the recent fibre-frenzy, it's been forgotten that fibre in itself doesn't help us lose weight: it only does that by helping us to reduce our intake of fat and sugar. It's certainly true, though, that increasing our intake of fibre does have other beneficial effects – it may also have a couple of minor drawbacks, but we can counteract these.

Fibre, as we've seen, is a form of carbohydrate, but it's 'unavailable' carbohydrate because we can't digest it. It's present in all plants and helps to give them their structure. In fact, it's fibre that fulfils the same function in plants as bones do in animals – it stops them becoming a heap of jelly on the floor. Fibre provides the structural support which helps plants stand upright. There are two types of fibre – soluble and insoluble.

Insoluble fibre is found mostly in cereals – like wheat and therefore flour – and also in fibrous fruit and vegetables. Fibre used to be called 'roughage' – though in fact 'smoothage' would be a better word, because this sort of fibre helps food and waste products pass smoothly through our digestive system. It increases the rate at which this happens and so helps to prevent constipation. Food rich in insoluble fibre needs more chewing and then when it reaches the stomach tends to absorb water and to swell a little – both these things tend to make us feel full and satisfied after a fibre-rich meal.

Soluble fibre is present in fruits, vegetables and pulses like lentils, peas and beans. Soluble fibre again absorbs water in the stomach and forms a gel. Then it delays the absorption of some nutrients from food. This is an advantage because it slows the absorption of sugar from the gut into the bloodstream. If we eat a large quantity of sugar without fibre, it causes a big rise in the sugar level in the blood and this is followed later by an equally large fall, which makes us feel hungry. So the advantage of this type of fibre is that it helps prevent hunger between meals.

Too little fibre

One of the problems with the average British diet is that we're not eating enough fibre. Apart from the serious medical conditions associated with a low-fibre diet which are outlined below, this lack of fibre leaves us with room in our tummies for those fatty sugary foods which make us fat. The average British diet at the moment contains just over $\frac{2}{3}$ oz (20g) of fibre a day. This is very low compared with, for example, rural Africans whose intake is between 2 and 4½ oz (50 and 120 g) of fibre a day. During the Second World War, 1¼ to 1½ oz (32–40 g) of fibre a day was the average intake and at present vegetarians in the UK consume 1½ oz (42 g) a day on average. The consensus of medical opinion is that we should be eating at least 1¼ oz (30 g) of fibre a day – 50 per cent up on our present intake. You'll be doing this on the BBC Diet *and* losing weight.

Fibre and health

Many diseases which are common in the western world are associated with a lack of fibre in the diet; these diseases are rare in communities which eat a high fibre diet.

- *Constipation.* About 40 per cent of the British population think they are constipated and about 20 per cent take laxatives. The benefits of a diet higher in fibre in treating constipation are now clear – and it's healthier and cheaper than taking laxatives.
- *Diverticular disease.* This is a disease of the large bowel which is characterised by small pouches in the wall of the bowel which can become inflamed. It's believed to be associated with a low-fibre diet, and increasing the fibre in the diet relieves the symptoms.
- *Cancer of the large bowel.* Development of this cancer is favoured by a low-fibre diet and there's good evidence that increasing the fibre in our diet may help to prevent it.
- *Heart disease.* A high level of cholesterol in the blood contributes to the furring-up of arteries which is the foundation for heart attacks and strokes. A diet high in fibre helps to reduce the level of cholesterol in the blood and so reduce the risk of a heart attack.
- *Diabetes* is very uncommon in communities with diets high in fibre and increasing the fibre in our diet may reduce our risk of developing it.
- *Gall-stones* tend to form more easily when the diet is lacking in fibre.
- *Other diseases* where a low-fibre diet is implicated include:
  appendicitis
  haemorrhoids (piles)
  hiatus hernia
  varicose veins

Fibre and losing weight

We've already seen some of the ways in which increasing the amount of fibre in our diet can help us to lose weight. Here's a checklist of those ways, plus one other.

- Fibre-rich foods are filling but not fattening, weight-for-weight. They don't fill us with too many calories in relation to the satisfaction they give.
- Fibre-rich foods tend to take longer to chew, which helps to satisfy hunger; once in the stomach they tend to swell a little helping us to feel full.
- Fibre-rich foods help to slow down the rate at which we absorb sugar from our food into the bloodstream. As there's no surge of sugar going into the bloodstream, the body doesn't react by issuing a surge of insulin which would lead to a high blood sugar level being followed by a low blood sugar level – causing hunger between meals. Instead, the levels of blood sugar tend to be more steady and to fluctuate less.
- Fibre-rich foods, for all these reasons, will help us to lose weight by cutting down our fat and sugar intakes far more easily and effortlessly than would otherwise be the case. The calories we take in by increasing fibre-rich foods are still far fewer than the calories we would take in from fat and sugar.
- Fibre-rich foods may also help slimmers in another, and perhaps surprising way. Whatever food we eat, we don't absorb all the calories it contains. For one thing, our digestive systems are not 100 per cent efficient and a few of the calories – perhaps 5–10 per cent – pass straight through. The other thing is that some of the calories potentially present in the food are 'unavailable' to us because we don't possess the necessary enzymes to break that type of food down (grass contains nourishing calories for cows, for example, but not for us!). Fibre itself comes into this 'unavailable' category – and calorie charts, by the way, have already taken this unavailability factor into account.

There's evidence now that fibre-rich foods may help to reduce the amount of energy, the number of calories, that our digestive system can absorb from food. This is not yet fully understood, but if it's true it's an additional bonus which will help us lose weight more easily on the BBC Diet.

Are there any drawbacks to fibre?

There are two drawbacks to fibre, and the first is connected with that last beneficial point.

- As well as the possibility of blocking the absorption of some unwanted calories, it seems that a large amount of fibre may interfere with the absorption of some wanted and needed minerals. Iron and calcium are the two most important minerals that are involved. People who have really gone over the top in increasing the amount of fibre that they eat may have had some problems here. The BBC Diet has two safeguards, though. Firstly, although the amount of fibre you eat will increase by following the Diet, it shouldn't be great enough to cause these problems. Secondly, you'll be getting enough iron and calcium anyway. There will be sufficient iron in meat and vegetables, especially green leafy ones; and the vitamin C from fresh fruit and vegetables will help your body absorb the iron it needs. And you'll be getting enough calcium in ½ pint (300 ml) of skimmed milk a day, leaving aside the extra calcium from other foods.
- Some fibre-rich foods, particularly pulses, peas and beans, cause gas to be produced in the intestines. (Gas is, of course, normally produced in the intestines – about a couple of pints a day.) This gas has to go somewhere of course and it may give you flatulence – wind up or down! As your body adjusts to the higher fibre in your diet, this problem will disappear. But if it's causing you a lot of bother, you could reduce the amount of peas and beans you eat and then increase gradually. Throwing away the soaking water of dried peas and beans and cooking them in fresh water will help too. This should be only a minor problem and a temporary one. If it really is a nuisance for you, remember there are many other sources of fibre other than peas and beans.

You can now see why the BBC Diet is based on these three principles:

- reducing fat
- reducing sugar
- increasing fibre

With these three principles and the further one of starting to take exercise, this is the diet which has the latest scientific and medical facts behind it to back it up and help you lose weight!

CHAPTER 5

ALL THOSE DIETS

You now know the principles on which a healthy diet *has* to be based and we'll soon be putting those principles into practice.

But what about all the conflicting advice that's still around? What about all those other diets? What about other ways of losing weight: diet foods, tablets, clubs, injections, surgery? What about those methods which abolish food and instead give you a slug of chemicals?

This chapter gives you the lowdown on the slimming industries and how weight loss really happens. I think the very best way to lose weight is by keeping control of your own body and your own health and by continuing to eat food that you enjoy – exactly the method of the BBC Diet. I hope at the end of this chapter that you think so too.

THERE'S ONLY ONE WAY TO LOSE WEIGHT

It's true: there *is* only one way to lose weight: you have to get into a 'negative energy balance'. The energy you take in (as food) has to be less than the energy you use (in just staying alive and in exercise). When that happens, your body is forced to use some of its stored energy – most of which is fat. As long as you are in an energy deficit, your body will keep drawing on its energy reserves and you'll lose weight. If you understand this, you'll understand how weight can be lost and you can never be conned.

It's difficult to calculate what the average calorie intake is in this country; methods based on asking people what they had to eat the day before are notoriously unreliable. But there is a National Food Survey which uses the information from a large number of households which keep records of food consumed. On this basis, the average energy intake is 2250 calories a day. Of course, some people are eating half this number and others are perhaps eating double it. (One of the question marks over its accuracy is that it only measures food consumed inside the home; as we know, the amount of food eaten outside the home has been increasing.)

To lose weight at a steady and reasonable rate (see later in this chapter) men need to reduce their intake to about 1500 calories a day and women to about 1250, and both need to increase their amount of physical activity. Some small, particularly inactive, women may need to reduce their calories to 1000 a day in order to lose weight at a reasonable rate. With the BBC Diet, you'll automatically reduce your calorie intake to between 1200 and 1500 calories a day (depending how strictly you follow the guidelines) by reducing your fat and sugar consumption. You'll see later in the book exactly how to do this and there are also set plans which are designed so that the calorie intake is about 1000, 1250 and 1500 if you want to follow this method (see Chapter Seven). As exercise is an integral part of the BBC Diet, you'll not only be reducing your calorie intake but also be speeding up the rate at which you burn calories, so your weight loss will be even greater and faster.

'MAGIC DIETS'

I could invent any number of diets which, if followed to the letter, would *guarantee* weight loss. Here are a couple of starters:

‹‹ **Tuna and Cucumber Diet** Eat five cans of tuna fish a day (packed in brine, not oil) and as much cucumber as you like – and nothing else – for two weeks. You'll be astounded at your weight loss, I promise! ››

‹‹ **The Egg and Lettuce Diet** Eat ten eggs (size 3) a day and as much lettuce as you like (pounds and pounds, if you want) – and nothing else – for two weeks. Your friends will be astounded at the new you – and that's a promise! ››

Are they beginning to sound familiar? I'm not for one moment suggesting that you follow one of these 'diets' – that would be not only unhealthy but also boring. But if you were to do so, you would assuredly lose weight. How do I know for certain? Well, what you would have done would have been to reduce drastically your calorie, or energy, intake. Even if you really worked hard at the cucumbers and lettuce – and I'm talking about double figures for each – you'd be hard pushed to reach a consumption level of 1000 calories a day. And this is presuming you'd get through the five tins of tuna or the ten eggs!

This is one way of cutting calories: the 'magic' two or three foods which will miraculously help you to lose weight provided you stick to them and nothing else. All you're doing *is* cutting calories – the hard way. If you stick to just a couple of foods like this, you can't help but cut calories and so lose weight. But it's difficult, boring and abnormal – and unnecessary. Don't believe any diet that tells you that if you stick to grapes and grapefruit, pineapple and papayas these will have strange effects (hitherto unknown to science) that help you burn off fat. It's a con: if they work at all, you'll know you've just been cutting those calories. Remember that losing weight depends on the food that you *don't* eat, not on the food that you *do*.

Here's another variation on the calorie-cutting con. Eat as much as you like – and lose weight. The snag is, it's as much as you like of one food. Often these sort of diets are handed round by friends on photocopied sheets. Here's a typical sales pitch:

    ❝ Enormous weight loss with the Bamboo-Shoot Diet. Eat as many Bamboo-shoots as you like – nibble it all day long – stuff yourself with it – the pounds will drop off **❞**

Again, I'm sure this would work. But we're talking about serious bamboo-shoot eating here! You'd have to manage about 12 lb (5.5 kg) of the stuff to reach 1000 calories – you'd never be able to reach that amount so again you would lose weight on what would be a semi-starvation diet. That's dangerous. This sort of diet, by the way, often favours exotic and expensive ingredients: the 'raw cabbage diet' would work as well but not sound quite so convincing – again you'd have to eat about 12 lb (5.5 kg) of cabbage to begin to approach 1000 calories.

These sort of diets rely on the monotony principle; it's been shown that with a very limited range of food it's easier to take in less and therefore reduce calories than when eating a wide variety of food. Appetite – determining the sort of food we fancy eating – as well as sheer hunger plays a part in the amount of food we eat.

The most that could be said about diets of this kind is that they would be effective in cutting calories – but although you do have to do that to lose weight, it's not, as we shall see, the whole story.

But diets of this kind should **never** be followed:

- because they are dangerous. Just eating one or two kinds of food is not a safe way to slim; remember your body doesn't need only calories from food but other nutrients too.

● because, ultimately, they are not effective. Eating pounds of tuna or bamboo-shoots doesn't help you when you go back to a normal life after your diet. You haven't done anything to tackle the eating habits which got you fat in the first place.

In effect, as I've said, these sorts of diets are semi-starvation ones. There are other semi-starvation diets around (rather more expensive ones) or very low-calorie diets which were formulated to meet the first criticism above. They are a more balanced formula, giving, the manufacturers claim, all the nutrients the body requires while drastically reducing calorie intake. We'll be considering them later in this chapter.

But why all this fuss and expense? If you are really desperate to lose weight, why not just go the whole hog and starve yourself completely? Why not force the body to use up its fat store for the purpose it was presumably put there for in the first place – to stop you starving to death when there's no food around? That this would be foolish and dangerous, I need hardly say; while total fasting takes some time to kill some people, others have died suddenly and unexpectedly while trying it. But, even more terrible, they would have died in vain, because total starvation is not even the most effective way to lose fat. Here's why:

WHAT DIET BOOKS NEVER TELL YOU

There's a difference between losing weight and losing fat. You can lose *weight* – perhaps ½ stone (3.5 kg) or so – in a few hours by sweating it out in a Turkish bath. But you won't have lost any *fat*. The key to sustained and permanent weight loss is losing fat; and even total starvation is not the most effective way of doing that. After all, your fat is there, so your body thinks, for a life or death purpose and it's not going to let it go easily.

Notice that all those extravagant claims in diet books – 'lose up to 20 pounds (9 kg) in 14 days' – don't tell you 20 pounds of what. It can't be fat: it's scientifically impossible. All diets which effectively cut calories will give you a rapid weight loss in the first couple of weeks – and the BBC Diet is no exception. But we don't make extravagant claims for it; to sustain and continue that weight loss you need to change some of the food habits which caused you to get fat. If you do that, you won't again have a dramatic weight loss as in those first two or three weeks, but you will steadily but surely slim down until you reach your ideal weight. This is common sense, but in many diet books, common sense flies out the window.

The pattern of weight loss on any diet which reduces calories to the safe minimum of 1000-1200 for women and 1200-1500 for men (which the BBC Diet does) is the same. Any variations are due to the way the individual body reacts to dieting (whether you're male or female, how fat you are, what sort of metabolism you have) and not, by and large, to the sort of diet you're following. The pattern is this:

The first 2 or 3 weeks	Rapid weight loss of between 7-21 lbs (3-9 kg)
The next 2 weeks	Weight loss of 2-4 lbs (1-2 kg) a week
The next month	Weight loss of 1-2 lbs (½-1 kg) a week

from then on the weight loss should be a steady 1-2 lbs (½-1 kg) a week until the ideal weight is reached.

Isn't starvation the ultimate diet?

If you think that this weight loss, after the initial rapid loss, doesn't sound spectular, consider this: after the initial rapid phase, the weight loss on a *total starvation* diet would only be about 4 lbs (2 kg) a week! This is the truth but most diet books don't tell you this as they want to sell diet books. Well, it's not that I don't want *this* book to sell, but I cannot tell you a lie. But here's the good news – a diet like the BBC Diet is actually more effective at promoting the loss of *fat* than total starvation.

On any diet, not all the weight loss is fat. The initial rapid weight loss occurs with all diets which have cut calories sufficiently – but most of this weight loss is *not* fat. The body stores its energy in three ways:

- One: as glucose in the bloodstream. This is immediately available and supplies, for example, the brain with the energy it needs to function.
- Two: as glycogen which is stored in the muscles and the liver. This can be made available very quickly.
- Three: as the fat stores themselves. This takes much longer for the body to start using. In starvation conditions, body tissue,

such as the protein in muscle, can also start being 'eaten up' to provide energy. It would be marvellous if we could say to our bodies 'I'm dieting; please just burn up fat', but unfortunately we can't!

The initial weight loss is, in fact, mostly water as glycogen is used up, water is released and the distribution of water in our body changes. (This water loss is different from the water sweated out in a Turkish bath: we don't gain the weight again if we drink extra water, as we would if it was just sweated out.)

This is true of all diets, no matter what they may extravagantly claim to the contrary. It doesn't mean that this initial phase isn't useful – you've lost weight, but not yet fat and it's a good morale boost at the beginning of a diet. But you shouldn't be misled by it. Nor be discouraged that subsequent weight loss is slower. Remember that this is inevitable; your body can't be forced to go as fast as in that initial phase, no matter which diet you're on – even if you were on a total starvation, zero-calorie diet. What will happen afterwards is that you begin to lose appreciabale fat as well as weight.

Even now though, all the weight loss is not fat. Unavoidably, you're also going to lose some protein from your lean tissue. Obviously, you want to keep this to the very minimum as you want to lose fat, not muscle. This is why – apart from its other dangers – total starvation is not the most effective way of losing fat. When you starve completely, about half the weight loss is not fat, but lean tissue. On a diet of 1000 calories, though, three-quarters of the weight you are losing is fat and only one quarter is lean tissue. This is obviously a far more desirable state of affairs, even if it is taking longer.

There's another reason for not being too drastic in dieting. We saw on page 17 how the body's natural response to a diet is to lower the basal metabolic rate (BMR) and so not burn up as many calories. The more drastic the diet, the greater the loss of lean, non-fat tissue which in turn causes the BMR to slow down even more proportionately. This is a vicious cycle as the body desperately tries to conserve its energy stores. It also means that it's a battle against the body which you'll find increasingly difficult to win. This is why it's much better to settle for a slower, but steady and safer weight loss.

One other point in the BBC Diet's favour: the old-fashioned

diets which were low in carbohydrates tended to lose more lean tissue than high-carbohydrates diets like the BBC's which tend to conserve the body's protein.

Getting food in proportion

Diets differ from one another in two ways: in the amount of calories they contain, and in the proportions of the different foodstuffs that they recommend make up these energy-reduced diets.

As our food consists basically of protein, fat and carbohydrate, it's the proportions of these three items that vary. If it is recommended that one item is increased, then it follows that one or more of the others must be decreased.

Amount of protein

There was a vogue some time ago for high protein diets. Invariably they also recommended decreasing carbohydrate and sometimes increasing fat. It's now known that these principles are scientifically unsound. The problems with high protein diets are:

- much of the protein we eat (for example in meat, milk and cheese) is bound up with saturated fat, so unrestricted protein diets will also unhealthily increase our intake of saturated fat
- they are low in dietary fibre
- high protein diets are not the most effective in promoting weight loss

Remember, that our protein intake has remained about the same over the last 50 years and at the moment in this country we eat, on average, about twice as much protein as we need. All nutritional and medical guidelines for healthy eating say that the amount of protein we eat should remain about the same. With the BBC Diet, we concentrate on low-fat but high quality protein sources such as lean meat, skinless chicken and white fish and also on proteins from cereals, vegetables and pulses.

Amount of fat

It's almost incredible to think now that anyone should recommend a high-fat diet as a means of losing weight – but books advocating just such a diet are still on sale. Of course, they usually say that they're cutting out carbohydrates, but that just means the proportion of energy from protein and fat rises, giving you a high-fat diet. High-fat diets are really bad news for your health: there is no doubt that if you carried on eating a diet like this you would shorten your life. If they can kill you in the long term, what damage can they be doing you in the short term? Unless you want to commit slow suicide, high-fat diets are out.

- Remember a diet high in saturated fats pushes up the level of cholesterol in your blood and increases the risks of heart attack and strokes.
- Weight for weight, fat contains twice as many calories as other foods; it's totally illogical to eat fats if you want to lose weight.
- Apart from their calorie content, there are other, metabolic reasons, why high-fat diets are not the most effective in losing weight.

The BBC Diet is a low-fat diet; the very best and most effective way to slim quickly and healthily. However, it doesn't try to cut out fats completely – some fat in the diet is essential for health and for making food palatable. There is at least one diet around which is ultra-low in fat and ultra-high in carbohydrates: it cuts out milk, eggs and cheese and limits meat and fish to about 3½ oz (90 g) a day. People other than vegetarians would find it difficult to follow and anyway there's no evidence that, for our health's sake, we need to be so drastic in cutting out the fat from our diet.

Amount of carbohydrate

This is the area in which a great deal of confusion used to reign in diet circles, and in one or two circles the confusion is still there. Sugar was correctly identified as 'fattening' (that is, having a high energy-density or many calories for a small amount) but all other carbohydrates were lumped in with it – so bread, potatoes, rice and pasta became classified as 'fattening' foods. We know now that we need to make a very important distinction between 'simple' or refined carbohydrates like sugar and 'complex' or unrefined ones like wholemeal bread and potatoes (see page 31). If we want to lose weight, we should certainly try to exclude sugar from our diet; we could banish every ounce of it and all we would cut out would be unwanted calories. But unrefined, complex carbohydrates can actually help us in losing weight.

There are still low-carbohydrate diets around which

confuse the two things and encourage us to eat fattening fat instead of filling but not fattening starches and fibres. Don't be misled!

Also, as we know, high-fibre diets are now in vogue and these are well attuned to modern nutritional thinking. Fibre isn't a magic pill though; it will only help us to lose weight if we also reduce fat and sugar – which is exactly what the BBC Diet does.

Increasing unrefined carbohydrates, increasing fibre and cutting out sugar is a far better way to lose weight than those low-carbohydrate diets.

- Eating more unrefined carbohydrates can help us lose weight in many ways, including helping us painlessly to reduce fat and sugar and helping us to feel full (see page 34).
- There's evidence that a high unrefined carbohydrate diet is the most effective way to slim; also that such a diet promotes the loss of the fat we want to lose and protects against the loss of lean tissue that we don't.
- It's also the very healthiest way to slim; you'll not only lose weight but also help to cut your risk of a wide range of diseases (see page 33).

Very low-calorie diets

These are currently fashionable and are marketed as the ideal way to lose weight. You don't need to think about food or calories at all, but just mix with water the chemicals the manufacturers sell to you and replace all your meals with them. They provide between 330 and 420 calories a day and, the makers claim, all essential nutrients. A government committee (COMA, reporting to the DHSS) has published a report about very low-calorie diets (VLCDs). It came to the conclusion that,

there is no evidence that VLCD regimes are more likely to achieve enduring weight loss than conventional weight-reducing diets, nor that they are more or less likely to be followed by weight regain than conventional diets. Claims for superiority in these respects over other diets are at present unsupported by valid data.

I take that to mean that VLCDs are a waste of your hard earned money! Isn't there something repulsive, too, about taking a chemical concoction rather than real food; food is not only the enemy with VLCDs but is totally annihilated. VLCDs do nothing to help you change unhealthy and fattening eating habits – which, even the manufacturers admit, is the key to keeping weight off once you've lost it.

The vast majority of people who are overweight are not ill (though they increase their risk of some diseases). These regimes treat you as if you are, cutting you off from life – meals out and sharing meals with family and friends – for weeks at a time. Just because you're overweight, you don't need to punish yourself so much.

It has to be said that for people who are grossly overweight – and I mean the people who can't get through doors – then, when other methods have failed, VLCDs may have a place in their treatment. But it is better anyway that they should be treated in specialised hospital obesity clinics.

The COMA report also recommends that people who are overweight should always try conventional weight-reducing diets first and then strongly recommends that they check with their doctors before they start to use a VLCD diet. If the use of the VLCD is prolonged beyond a few weeks, then the report states that medical supervision is required.

In the 1970s, when VLCDs began to be marketed commercially, the United States Food and Drug Administration introduced regulations which stated that liquid protein diets should bear the following warning, 'very low calorie protein diets (below 400 kcal a day) may cause serious illness or death. Do not use this weight reduction without medical supervision. Not for use by infants, children or pregnant or nursing women.'

The subsequent development of VLCDs has sought to meet the dangers in the early preparations by changing their formulation and providing high quality protein and a different protein-to-carbohydrate ratio and by including the complete range of minerals and vitamins. Nevertheless, the manufacturers still advise people to consult their doctors before starting a VLCD. Ask yourself this question: 'do I need to consult my doctor before eating a meal?'

OTHER WAYS OF LOSING WEIGHT

Slimming Clubs

Some people find they do get encouragement and motivation from being with other people in the same situation and from being able to share and discuss problems. Many people slim successfully by themselves, but if you feel you'd get disheartened, you may find a slimming club helpful. There are clubs run by large national chains and also some local authorities run them. Beware of extravagant claims of slimming clubs though. It's difficult fully to assess their performance on a long-term basis – remember you could do equally well yourself.

If you do go to a slimming club, check that the diet they suggest you follow will be effective and healthy. Check that it's a diet low in fat, low in sugar and high in complex carbohydrates, starches and fibre. Also check that the club gives you advice about weight maintenance by following the same principles of healthy eating.

Of course, if you don't want to slim on your own, another way of following the BBC Diet is to invite some friends to follow it with you.

Drugs and tablets

There are tablets you can buy over the counter which claim to help weight loss and there are ones that your doctor can prescribe for you.

The ones you buy over the counter are sold as appetite reducers. These are of several types but one of the most popular consists of methyl cellulose which is said to reduce hunger by providing bulk, swelling up in the stomach and so decreasing appetite. But the products on sale contain only small amounts of methyl cellulose and so there is no evidence that they are an effective means of reducing food intake. You may remember that fibre in your food works in the same way and really is effective.

Other tablets contain glucose and claim that if taken before a meal they reduce your appetite. You'd probably find that eating an apple before a meal would have the same effect.

Drugs that doctors can prescribe are more effective. They reduce appetite but they also have side effects. They are therefore not recommended in minor degrees of overweight, but only where there is a substantial risk to health. This is something your doctor would decide, but for most people who are overweight, the side effects would far outweigh the benefits.

Surgery

This is resorted to only in very severe cases and when all other methods of treatment have failed. The simplest is wiring the jaws together so that only liquid can be drunk, but more drastically, part of the stomach may be removed or part of the intestine may be bypassed. These are extreme measures, and, of course, are only undertaken for the very few enormously obese people whose life is in immediate danger.

'Miracles'

People who are really very anxious about being fat and who are desperate to lose weight are at the mercy of all kinds of conmen. 'There must be some tablet or injection or machine that can help', they think; and many embrace, expensively, the latest 'miracle' as it comes along.

There is no miracle: if there were, it would be available on the NHS as, I assure you, doctors have no vested interest in people being fat and would welcome with open arms a quick cure for obesity.

Neither grapefruits, nor pineapples, nor Bai-lin tea nor massage, nor electrical currents can melt one ounce of fat away. Beware of *anything* that costs you money to lose weight – with the possible exception of slimming clubs if you would find them useful. Losing weight is free – if you're determined to do it. There's no mystery about it. You cut down your calories and increase your exercise. Here's how in the following chapters.

CHAPTER 6

THE BBC DIET-THE FIRST STEP: MOTIVATION AND PREPARATION

There are people with iron self-discipline who, once they have decided on a course of action, can begin it and follow it through to the end. They can skip this chapter completely and go to Chapter Seven and begin the BBC Diet.

I expect most of you are still with me – like me, you haven't got iron self-discipline. If there's something I have to do – like writing a book! – I have to psyche myself up for it, motivate myself to do it, prepare to do it – and then jump in and do it. Even when I'm doing it, I have to keep myself going telling myself that it's something I should be doing, I need to do, I'll feel so good when I've finished it. Sound familiar? Most of us go through similar processes in all sorts of areas of our life, from mowing the lawn to writing out our Christmas cards. If you smoke and wanted to stop, you'd be more likely to be successful if you went through a similar process. And so it is with dieting and that's what this chapter is about – motivating yourself and planning and preparing so that you'll have the best possible chance of success.

Read this chapter and then do the things it suggests which sound right for you. Not everything will be right for everybody – but there'll be some things here which will help *you* enormously in shedding those pounds.

WHAT SORT OF PERSON ARE YOU?

This requires an honest assessment! Although everyone following the BBC Diet will be doing the same basic things, how you personally follow it will be crucial to your success. You've got to get your own personality on your side in helping you win and not fight against your own nature. The secret of happiness, or success, in this as in all things, is accepting yourself for what you are and then working on how you live with yourself!

- Are you the kind of person who likes to keep rules – or do you rebel against them? Some diet books (often, I blush to say, written by doctors) have RULES carved on tablets of stone.

  'Eat 5 oz of grilled haddock at 12.45 pm every Wednesday.'
  'What if I'm out working or I can only get cod?'
  'No swaps are allowed – you will only lose weight if you stick to this diet to the letter.'

  You know the sort of thing. It's treating people who want to slim as children or feeble-minded. It's not the order you eat food in or the time you eat it that makes you lose weight – it's the food you don't eat and the calories you cut down on. It has to be said, though, that some people do like order. If you are one of those, then the prescription I give for you to lose weight is to follow *exactly* one of our dieting plans; don't deviate by one radish. For you, this is the very best possible way to follow the BBC Diet.

- If you don't like blindly following rules, you can learn and understand the guidelines and then apply them to whatever situation you find yourself in. This is again relatively easy, but it has to be right for your personality

  I suspect that, in this matter, most of us will be somewhere in the middle, and will roughly follow a plan, but use our commensense to tell us when and how we can adapt it to meet the circumstances in which we live. Again, the BBC Diet tells you how to build in that flexibility.

- Does 'moderation' work for you? Some people can follow a diet fairly strictly for most of the time, deviate from it and then get right back on it. For example you may be offered a piece of someone's birthday cake and you can't refuse, or you go out for a meal on your wedding anniversary and your absolutely favourite, fattening dish is on the menu. It's not a sin to say, 'For the next five minutes or the next three hours, I'm off my diet.' All you will have done, if you immediately go right back to following your diet, is to slow your weight loss down by a tiny, insignificant fraction. So what?

  Make sure you *are* that sort of person, though – and not the sort of person who ends up saying 'I'm off my diet for five minutes' several times a day! If you pretend you're the first sort of person and are actually the second, it's all going to end in tears. Believe me, you know what sort of person you are.

On the other hand, you may be another sort, who accepts that one chocolate and then thinks 'Oh, I knew I couldn't diet' and proceeds to eat a whole box.

If you're either of these last two, moderation is *not* for you and you'll have to be firm with yourself.

- Do you have to have a fast result or can you live with slow but steady progress knowing that you will reach your goal eventually? In other words, is the only way to success for you to stick to a diet until you've reached your ideal weight, or can you afford to be more flexible and think, 'I'll diet for two weeks, then enjoy myself – but still eat fairly sensibly for another two – and then go back on my diet for another two'. This is a great way to lose weight if you can do it and are prepared to wait a couple of months for a result rather than a few weeks. But again, beware you're not the sort of person who, once the first bout of dieting is over, never goes back on it again and forgets all about the ideal weight that you were trying to reach.
- Am I scrupulously honest with myself or do I cheat a little? If you cheat and pretend to yourself that you're not eating what in fact you are eating, then you won't lose weight at the rate you hoped for. If you don't cheat too much, you'll still lose weight. It's fine if you do cheat as long as you admit it; then you won't be disappointed when your weight loss isn't quite as fast as you expected. You then have to ask yourself the question, 'Would I rather feel free to cheat a little or lose weight faster?' The correct option is the one you're happy with.

Motivation

Of course, you're motivated to lose weight: otherwise you wouldn't be reading this book. But it's important to think of your reasons and to write them down. You'll find this a great help in becoming enthusiastic about getting started – and keeping you enthusiastic if you begin to wane in the middle of your diet. Write down your reasons and make sure you keep the piece of paper or book you write them in. Of course, your reasons are particular to you, but some of them could be variations of the following:

- It's my daughter's wedding in the summer and I want to look good for that

- We're going to Greece in July and I want to appear on the beach without blushing
- I want to get into a size 10 dress again
- I want to get into my best blue suit for our wedding anniversary
- My wife/husband would like me to be slimmer
- I feel I'll be sexier if I'm slimmer
- I want girls to say 'yes' when I ask them to dance
- I don't want to be out of breath when playing with my grandchildren
- I want to ease the pain of the arthritis in my knees
- I want to reduce my risk of a heart attack (not a very good selling point this last one, I admit – but true though!)

The only reasons that will be powerful and motivating for you will be your own. Try to think of and write down at least ten of them. It doesn't matter if they sound rather silly or 'unworthy' – this isn't an exam and you don't need to show them to a living soul.

Enlisting help

Use your family and friends to help you to slim. If you're married, it's vital that you get your husband or wife to help you. Perhaps if your spouse is a little on the podgy side, you could slim together – that will certainly make it easier. If your spouse is unhelpful and says, 'I like you the way you are' then talk about some of the reasons you want to slim and explain, tactfully, that *you'd* feel much happier if you lost some weight.

Some people find it useful to slim with a friend – you can compare notes and support each other. You may or may not find it helpful to be competitive (hopefully your personalities will match in this respect) but on the whole it's probably better not to be, but rather to encourage and so reinforce each other's success.

You will also find it a good idea to let family and friends know not only that you are slimming, but also how much weight you're hoping to lose. Then you should give them progress reports. This may begin to bore them, but if at least they seem to be enthusiastic this will give you another boost. On the other hand, your personality may be such that you'd rather tell no one, slim in secret and wait for unsolicited comments. Again, do what suits you best.

Contracts and rewards

Signing a contract or pledge with yourself or with someone else, promising to lose weight and rewarding yourself or being rewarded for losing weight might sound rather alien and 'UnBritish'! But if you think about it, we operate a system of contracts and rewards with ourselves all the time in minor and major ways, consciously or only half-consciously.

If I'm writing something, for example, I might spur myself on by saying to myself, 'I'll just finish this section and then I'll have a cup of tea.' That's a contract and a reward. I could have just had the cup of tea immediately, but what I did was make a contract, 'I'll finish this section,' and after I'd finished it give myself the reward, a cup of tea. So, I had something pleasant to look forward to when I finished the less pleasant task, and the cup of tea helped to reinforce my 'good' behaviour, finishing the section. This might sound rather far-fetched, but it is one of the little tricks that we play with ourselves all the time in order to accomplish things that we really want to do, but could easily get distracted from and not get done.

'I'll clean the oven, then I'll read the paper.'

'I'll mow the lawn, then I'll have a glass of lager.'

'I'll wash the dishes, then I'll put my feet up.'

'I'll work all year, and then I'll have a fortnight on a sunny beach.'

This last one is different from the rest as the reward isn't immediate. Here we have to use our imagination: longing for that warm sun and sand through the short cold days of January and February. Losing weight is more like this. You know there's going to be a reward, but it's a little time coming. In the meanwhile, a bar of chocolate beckons which offers immediate satisfaction. You have constantly to remind yourself that that chocolate takes your ultimate reward of being slim further away.

So some people, again not all, find it very useful while following a diet to have both a written contract and intermediate rewards for specific achievements along the road to reaching their goal. You need to write this down so that you can look at it now and again, along with your reasons for slimming, which will be particularly useful in times of temptation.

The contract could just be with yourself, for example:

I, TONY ANDREWS,

promise myself that I shall lose
15 lb (6.75 kg) in weight.

After losing the first 5 lb (2.25 kg) I shall buy myself
a Barbara Dickson cassette.

After losing the next 5 lb (2.25 kg) I shall buy myself
a set of fishing floats and weights.

And after losing the whole 15 lb (6.75 kg) I shall buy myself
a new suit.

Present Weight: 13 st 8 lb   Signed: Tony Andrews
Target Weight: 12 st 7 lb   Date: ....

Alternatively, and better, the contract could be with your spouse, another member of your family, or a friend. For example:

I, Liz Andrews, promise that I shall
lose 1½ stone (11 kg) in weight
and I, Tony Andrews, promise to
support and help her.
After she has lost ½ stone (3.5 kg) I shall give
her three breakfasts (healthy and slimming)
in bed.

After she has lost a further ½ stone (3.5 kg)
I shall pay for her to have her hair done
and after she has lost the whole 1½ stone (11 kg)
I shall buy her a new dress.

Present Weight: 10 st 8 lb   Signed: Liz Andrews
Target Weight: 9 st   Tony Andrews
              Date: ....

- It might also be useful to pin a full-length photograph of yourself on the contract so that you remember why you want to lose weight; imagining the new you is then a futher 'reward'.
- It's best to give rewards for progress – losing 2 or 5 lb (1 or 2 kg) – as well as for reaching a target weight.
- If you're quite a bit overweight, don't make your target weight as low as your ideal weight: you may get discouraged if progress is slower than you had hoped. Once you've reached one target weight, you can set yourself another and have a new contract.
- Rewards do not have to be extravagant in order to be effective. Simple rewards like a lie-in, breakfast in bed, someone else doing the washing up, can all work well. On the other hand, if you can persuade your husband that the new slim you is worth a weekend in Paris. . . .
- Do I need to say that rewards of boxes of chocolates are OUT!
- Some people may feel that the threat of punishment rather than a reward may work. For example you may give someone £1 a week and only get it back if and when you reach your target weight. Sounds tough to me, but something like this may work for you. Perhaps you could also get your friend or partner to match your £1 each time, so it's double or quits.

Watching your progress

At the minimum, it's useful to write down your present weight and then write in, with the date, your weight each week. Ideally, you should only weigh yourself once a week, at the same time of day on the same set of scales, and preferably with no clothes on – if not, then at least a similar set of clothes. I know, of course, you will ignore this and weigh yourself every day – or even twice a day! Remember though that our weight fluctuates because of water loss or retention on a day-to-day basis and the weekly figures will give you a much more accurate picture of the progress you're making. Remember also that your weight loss will be greater and faster at the beginning of the diet than later on: don't be discouraged by this, it's not only normal but inevitable. Remember that a loss of even 1 lb (roughly $\frac{1}{2}$ kg) a week would be $3\frac{1}{4}$ stone (24 kg) lighter in a year!

Some people may also find it useful to keep a note of their measurements as well as their weight. Do this every couple of weeks – or once a month if you can bear to wait. You may find it easier to get your spouse or a friend to take the measurements for you. You could use a chart like the one below or simply write notes on a piece of paper.

Date	Bust/ Chest	Waist	Hips	Thigh	Upper Arm

Keeping a food diary

Before you start slimming, it's useful to know what sort of food you are presently eating so that you can identify problem areas. If you know exactly the sort of food you're eating, you'll know what is helping to make you fat.

'Well, of course I know what I eat,' you may be saying – let me assure that you don't: no one does. Everyone, when asked to recount exactly what they had to eat the day before, is inaccurate, sometimes wildly so. We all forget the odd custard cream biscuit, the handful of peanuts, the toddler's leftover baked beans – food we often eat absentmindedly. By keeping a food diary before you start to slim, you'll get a much more accurate picture of what you're eating. Ideally, you should keep one for a week, but even a day or two will help. Remember that your pattern of eating at the weekend will be different from that during the week, so if you're only going to do two days, choose one weekday and one weekend day.

Your food diary could be done on any piece of paper. There's an example of how one might look on the page opposite.

You don't need to do it in quite as much detail, though it will only take you a few minutes if you do. The calories in that day were about 2800! Now go through your diary and see what you can learn from it.

DAY AND DATE

WHEN?	WHERE?	WHAT?	WITH WHOM?	ACTIVITY	HUNGRY?	MOOD	COMMENT
7.45 am	Bedroom	2 digestive biscuits 1 tea with sugar	Alone	Getting dressed	Not really	Rush	Didn't think about it
11.10 am	Office	1 doughnut 1 coffee with sugar	Catrin & Tessa	Writing	Yes	Bored	Wish I'd waited 'till lunch
12.45 pm	Canteen	2 sausages, chips & peas 1 tea with sugar	David & Tony	Talking	Yes	OK	More interested in the gossip than food
3.30 pm	Office	Cream cake 1 tea with sugar	6 people	Talking – John's birthday	No	OK	Difficult to say no to the cream cake
6.30 pm	Home	Cheese & onion sandwich (white bread) 1 tea with sugar	Family	Watching TV & talking	Yes	Tired	Eating without really noticing it
10.00 pm	Home	Glass of lager – 1 pkt crisps & 1 piece of pork pie	Husband	Watching TV	No	OK	Caught up in TV programme

- How can you cut down the fat and the sugar? In the example, you could have done so by not having sugar in tea or coffee; not having cakes or pastries – you could have had fruit instead; not having chips – you could have had a baked potato instead; not having high-fat pie and chips as a snack – instead having a proper meal, perhaps tuna fish salad, earlier. You could also have cut out the alcohol and had a low-calorie drink. You could have increased your fibre by having wholemeal breakfast cereal, the baked potato, and wholemeal bread with your tuna salad.
- Go through your diet diary and ask yourself about everything you eat. Does this contain fat or sugar? What could I have had to eat instead? How can I increase the fibre?
- Why did you eat when you weren't hungry? Are there times when you can cut calories by stopping unnecessary eating?
- How do you say no to cream cakes? If everyone knows you're trying to slim, this will be easier.
- How many times did you snack? You're much more likely to lose weight if you only eat at regular mealtimes, instead of 'nibbling' and 'picking' and 'eating on the move'. If you have to snack, make sure you do so on non-fattening foods like fruit and vegetables.
- How many times did you eat when you were also doing something else? If we're doing something like watching television, we can pile in food without even noticing it, let alone enjoying it. When you start slimming don't do anything else while you're eating.
- Did you eat when you were bored or unhappy? Eating for reasons other than hunger can really make us pile in extra calories.

Shopping

If you live on your own and you don't buy fatty sugary food, then you're already halfway to success. If you live with your family, you've got to develop other strategies as well (see below) but even then you should think carefully about how shopping wisely would help you with your slimming.

- Always write out a shopping list. That way you'll be less likely to make impulse purchases. When you've written your list go through it again, asking yourself, 'Is there any fatty, sugary food I can cross off?' and 'Can I think of a more slimming and healthy alternative for this?'

- Never shop on an empty stomach. You'll be at much greater risk then of making impulse purchases, which are likely to be fatty and sugary. I can confess that when I've been really hungry when shopping I've bought things like pork pies and scotch eggs and eaten them in the car park. I've even eaten a packet of crisps while walking round the supermarket and presented the empty bag at the check-out – something you've never done, I'm sure! Supermarkets want to tempt you with food, especially processed food, and you're most vulnerable when you're hungry.
- Beware of tricks that supermarkets play – like chocolate at the check-out. If you're aware of tricks, you're less likely to fall for them.
- Start looking at food labels. Food ingredients are listed in weight order, that is with the biggest single ingredient coming first. Again, think fat, think sugar. It's a very rare processed food that doesn't contain one of these, if not both.
- Avoid temptation. If you know you always buy cream cakes at the bakers because they're so delicious, start buying your bread from the supermarket.

Food and the family

As I've said, if you live alone and have no fattening food in the house, you can't be tempted by it. But a family isn't going to take too kindly to your not buying chocolate, jam tarts and crisps just because you're slimming. There are two strategies here.

- Make sure you also buy plenty of non-fattening snack alternatives for yourself – like fruit – so that you can't say 'I must eat something and there's nothing else in.'
- If you buy cream cakes, for example, buy only one each for the other members of the family. If you buy crisps for your son or daughter, put them in a paper bag with 'John's' or 'Janet's' on the side in big letters. If you have to buy chocolate biscuits for the family, wrap them up in several bags, so you've got more time for avoidance action if you are tempted.

The principles in this book don't just apply to slimmers – eating less fat and sugar and more fibre is healthier for everyone. So when you start slimming you can begin to change your whole family's diet to a more healthy one. This would also benefit you because you don't have to cook separate meals. The secret with changing a family's eating habits is to take it slowly. Don't cut out too many of their favourite foods all at once. For example, you could give them a healthy and low-fat main course, and apple pie and custard, or whatever they want, as a pudding. Meanwhile, you'll be having fresh fruit. When they insist on chips, you can have a baked potato, brown rice or pasta.

I know some dieters prefer to cook and eat separately from the rest of the family, but it's far easier to stick to a diet if you're eating at least some of the same food. It does make sense too, to think of their health as well as your figure.

CHAPTER 7

THE BBC DIET – THE SECOND STEP

So now you're ready to go. You know the reasons you've put on weight (from your food diary); you know why you want to lose weight (your ten reasons); and you've made a contract with yourself or someone else with some rewards for the progress you make. You're going to do it!

CHOOSE YOUR METHOD

There are two ways of following the BBC Diet. The first is by following one of the plans which come later in this chapter. These are designed to be flexible and you shouldn't find a problem in choosing one, or constructing your own in the ways suggested, so that it is easy to follow for the sort of life you lead. We also give you advice about eating out and entertaining.

The other way to follow the BBC Diet is by understanding and getting to know a series of guidelines, 'Where's the fat?', 'Where's the sugar?' and, 'Where's the fibre?'. On first sight, this method may seem rather hit and miss compared with some rigid diet plans you may have seen. But it's been shown that if you do follow the guidelines on cutting down fat and sugar – and apply them to every bit of food you eat – you will automatically cut down your calorie intake to between 1200 (following the guidelines strictly) to 1500 calories a day (following them a little more loosely), and this, of course, without counting calories. Increasing your fibre intake by following those guidelines will help you to cut down fat and sugar without feeling hungry.

The advantage of following guidelines as opposed to a set plan is clear: you're in control. In any situation – in a supermarket, in a restaurant, cooking for yourself or family or friends – you'll always know what to do to choose the slimming options. You won't need to carry around a plan which you continually have to refer to and may forget after a few weeks, but you'll have the knowledge for ever to enable you to stay slim and to stay healthy. In the long term, this really is the best idea – you won't be at the mercy of passing fad diets and you won't have to buy a slimming book again.

In practice, most people will probably use a mixture of the two methods. Some people will prefer to follow a set plan but will find the guidelines useful when they need greater flexibility and others will follow the guidelines but use parts of the set plans now and again to give them ideas and to make sure they're on the right lines.

Be realistic

It's very important not to be over ambitious and unrealistic in your goals. When you look through the guidelines and plans, be realistic about what you can achieve, and perhaps readjust your goal accordingly. It's much better to have one modest target, achieve that and then set yourself another and then perhaps another than have one large target, which may suddenly seem so far away that you give up altogether. If your goal is achieveable, then it's a considerable boost to further success if you attain it in a reasonable time.

I'm not, by the way, giving you a licence to fail, or to think that you won't reach your ideal weight – you will certainly do so if you're determined to, but reaching targets along the way will help enormously.

This is rather liberal talk for a Diet Book – as I've said before, many of them (usually written by doctors) are too authoritarian. 'Do not ever substitute'; 'if I say eat three slices of cucumber, then that is exactly what you should eat.' These doctors are well-meaning, but I am amazed at their lack of insight into human nature and their arrogance in thinking that their readers – and back in their surgery, their patients – will do exactly what they tell them.

It is not realistic to expect everyone to stick rigidly to a diet for weeks at a time. You may forget to buy something, you may have lunch out unexpectedly, friends may call round. This is why you need to be flexible; but you do need to understand the guidelines so your flexibility is 'safe' and you don't go undoing your good work.

There's another reason why I've wanted to stress realism and flexibility. Rigid, authoritarian diet plans may, as I've said, suit some people but in my view they can be unhelpful to many more because of one emotion they can induce: guilt. Guilt is not an appropriate emotion to have after eating a chocolate or a cream cake. Yet some people react as if it's a sin or a crime. So you've broken your diet – so what? You've just delayed reaching your ideal weight by a little. Put the past behind you, and just resolve to stick to your diet – from now on. You can only do something about your future meals and not your past ones.

THE BBC DIET GUIDELINES

Remember, we need to be aware of fat, sugar and fibre – in order to cut down the fat and sugar and increase the fibre.

Where's the fat?

Let's remind ourselves again where the fat comes from in the average British diet:

27 per cent from meat and meat products
25 per cent from butter and margarine
13 per cent from cooking oils and fats
13 per cent from milk
 6 per cent from biscuits, cakes and pastries
 5 per cent from cheese and cream
11 per cent from other foods

We'll consider how we cut down – or cut out – the fat in each of these categories. Remember that cutting down fat is the single most important thing we can do in our fight against the flab. Weight for weight, fat contains twice as many calories as protein and carbohydrate. We need to cut down our fat by as much as we can. How much is that? Read on.

Cutting down fat from meat and meat products

- Cut out meat products *completely*. This means things such as pies, pasties, sausages, pates, salami. All these are very high in fat; remember that fat is cheaper than meat and can be 'hidden' in these products. The only 'safe' meat is lean pieces that you can identify. If you don't want to cut out these products completely, look for the lower-fat versions of them.
- Cut off any visible fat on meat. Choose lean cuts, e.g. leg of lamb rather than shoulder. Your portion size of lean meat should be 2-3 oz (50-75 g).
- White chicken meat is very lean provided you remove the skin; this gets rid of most of the fat and half the calories. Again, your portion size should be 2-3 oz (50-75 g). Turkey and game are also low in fat; on the other hand duck and goose are quite fatty.

- Eat more fish. White fish is extremely low in fat. Portion size here can be 4-5 oz (100-150 g).

    Fish like herrings and mackerel contain more fat but grilled are not too high in calories. Choose canned fish like sardines and tuna packed in brine rather than oil – this almost halves the calories.
- Always grill rather than fry – this very significantly reduces the calories. Alternatively, microwave or poach in water or skimmed milk.
- If using mince, choose the leanest you can buy. Pour off all the fat after frying, or cover with water, bring slowly to the boil, simmer gently for a couple of minutes, pour off the now fatty water and then proceed with your recipe.
- In casseroles and other similar dishes you are making for yourself, cut down the amount of meat you would normally use. Remember even lean red meat has a significant fat content. To supplement the meat, add pulses like beans, lentils, split peas or chick peas.

Cutting down the fat from butter and margarine

- This fat is rather easier to identify and therefore avoid. Remember, on average, one quarter of the fat in our diet comes from these sources.
- Cut out butter and margarine as completely as you can.
- Substitute a low-fat spread such as Gold or Outline.
- Limit your intake of the low-fat spread to ½ oz (15 g) a day, (about two teaspoonfuls). Spread very thinly, this will just cover four slices of bread (yours will be wholemeal, of course). Alternatively, you could use ¼ oz (10 g) to cover two slices to make a sandwich and the other ¼ oz (10 g) could go into a baked potato. (I know you don't measure low-fat spread normally in teaspoonsful: if you scrape your knife tip very gently once across the packet, you'll end up with about ¼ oz or 10 g.) ½ oz (15 g) of low-fat spread, by the way, has about 50 calories; ½ oz (15 g) butter or margarine has about 100.
- Try making sandwiches with the low-fat spread on one slice of bread rather than both; if the filling is moist, try not adding any at all.

Cutting down the fat from cooking oils and fats

- You'll be cutting these down to the very minimum because you'll be grilling rather than frying.

- When you do want to fry, e.g. a chopped onion to begin a healthy pilaff or risotto, use a non-stick pan and you will find you can 'dry-fry' using no oil at all. Add a spoonful of water if it begins to stick, and stir all the time. Alternatively, you could use a very small amount of oil. You should be able to fry an onion in one-two teaspoonful of oil. This could, of course, be a dish for two-four people so the amount of oil per person will be very tiny. Low-fat spread is unsuitable for frying.
- One tablespoonful of oil is 120 calories. This is why you'll be measuring out your oil in teaspoonsful (40 calories) and certainly not pouring it from the bottle – one generous slurp could be a quarter of your calorie target for the day!
- For your health's sake and that of your family, use polyunsaturated oil rather than hard cooking fats or oils just labelled 'cooking oil'. Find a 'named' oil like sunflower, safflower or groundnut as these, particularly the first two, are high in polyunsaturates. Olive oil, which is also healthy (high in monounsaturates) is strongly flavoured and can therefore make its mark in a dish in very small quantities.
- Remember mayonnaise is largely oil and therefore packed with calories. Use low-fat natural yoghurt, thinned with a little wine vinegar, as a delicious alternative to both mayonnaise and vinaigrette or French dressing.
- When you're making chips for the family (and very occasionally for yourself when you've got to your ideal weight!) you can cut down the fat considerably. Cut your chips thickly (so that weight-for-weight there's a lower surface area to absorb the fat) and then fry them quickly in hot oil (hot oil seeps into the chips less than cooler oil). Again, use an oil high in polyunsaturates and don't keep re-using it (which causes it to become saturated fat). Finally, shake off as much oil as possible and then, before serving, drain the chips on kitchen paper to get rid of any remaining fat.

Cutting down the fat from milk

- This is easy: use only skimmed milk.
- Although ordinary (silver-top) milk seems fairly low in fat – it contains 4 per cent fat in fact – because we drink quite a lot of it, it contributes significantly to the total fat in our diet. If we drink just less than one pint (600 ml) of milk a day – 6 pints (3.5 litres) a week – then we would be consuming as much fat (and calories!) as in half a pint of double cream. Even $\frac{1}{2}$ pint

(300 ml) of milk a day is the equivalent of drinking a pint
(600 ml) of single cream a week.

- Semi-skimmed milk has half the fat of ordinary milk;
skimmed milk has virtually no fat at all. This is why
skimmed milk should be your choice: it contains only half
the calories of whole milk. It is thinner than whole milk but
you will soon get used to the taste. When you've reached
your ideal weight, you may be very happy staying with
skimmed milk and that would be excellent. If you do want
something a little richer, you could go to semi-skimmed
milk. Don't go back to whole milk.

- When you're trying to lose weight, you should aim to drink
½ pint (300 ml) of skimmed milk a day. This will give you
significant nutrients for less than 100 calories. In particular,
you'll be ensuring that you're getting enough calcium. You
should find that ½ pint (300 ml) is enough for your breakfast
cereal and cups of tea and coffee throughout the day.

Cutting down the fat from biscuits, cakes and pastries

- This is also easy to achieve: stop eating them. I know it's
easier to say than to achieve but it really will pay dividends if
you're trying to slim – at a stroke you wipe out this source
of fat in your diet.

- The other advantage of cutting this fat source is that it's all
here as sweet fat. You cut the fat and the sugar at the same
time.

- Fresh fruit is the healthy and slimming alternative to these
products.

Cutting down the fat from cream and cheese

- You know what to do about cream: it's a 'no-no' food while
you want to lose weight and very much a 'sometimes' food
once you've reached your ideal weight. Double cream is
48 per cent fat – that fact alone should stop you eating it.
Whipping cream is 35 per cent fat and single cream is 18 per
cent fat.

- There are tasty, healthy and low-fat substitutes for cream.
  □ low-fat natural yoghurt which is virtually fat free
  □ fromage frais or fromage blanc. This is a skimmed milk
  'cheese' though it isn't cheesy at all. It is delicious with
  fruit and it makes very good fruit fools. It comes in tubs
  of 1 per cent and 8 per cent fat varieties. You, of course,

will be choosing the 1 per cent (the 8 per cent has added cream).

□ Rather more calorific is Greek-style yoghurt which is 8-10 per cent fat or half the fat of single cream. This is all right as an occasional treat. The advantage of it is that you can add it to cooked dishes and, unlike low-fat natural yoghurt, it doesn't curdle. Adding one or two spoonfuls to a soup or a curry for two or four people is going to taste luxurious without adding too many calories. It may help to cut down the amount of cream the whole family eats. If you want to cook with low-fat natural yoghurt by the way, a teaspoonful of cornflour mixed with a little milk and stirred into it, will stabilise it.

- Some people regard cheese as a 'slimming' food. Let me assure you: it isn't. Cheddar-type cheeses are one-third fat. Stilton and cream cheeses are nearly half fat. One oz (25 g) of Cheddar cheese should be your portion while you want to lose weight. There are of course lower fat alternatives.

- Edam is always promoted as the slimmers' cheese. It is less full of fat than Cheddar – it's a quarter fat – but it's also, I think, rather bland. But it is cheap and some people find it delicious. Soft cheeses like Brie and Camembert are also about a quarter fat and are tastier. (The reason for the lower percentage fat content of soft cheeses compared with 'hard' cheese like Cheddar is that they contain more water – that's why they're soft! – and so contain less fat and fewer calories weight for weight.) Try still to stick to 1 oz (25 g) portions of soft cheeses – but you could go to 1½ oz (40 g) for the same calories as 1 oz (25 g) of Cheddar.

- There are now lower fat Cheddar-type cheeses on sale which usually contain less than half the fat of conventional Cheddar – they're about 14 per cent fat. Again, some of them taste rather bland but I have to say they seem to have greatly improved recently. There are also now many low-fat versions of soft cheeses. It's best to use all these products as a way of further cutting down your calories rather than a way of eating more cheese.

- Cottage cheese – the slimmer's friend! – is only 4 per cent fat. I have to say I'm not that keen on it, but if you like it, it's a great boon. I'm told (by Delia Smith, no less) that it's good stirred into mashed potatoes. That sounds a good idea if you don't add any other fat – you could always also add some skimmed milk.

- When using cheese in cooking, use less of a stronger flavoured variety – and perhaps add a little mustard.

Cutting down the rest of the fat in our diet This comes from a wide variety of sources but we only need to think about a few which are significant.

- Nuts and salted snacks, crisps and all those other strangely shaped objects, are high in fat. You need to cut them out completely while you're losing weight.
- Although eggs sometimes get a bad press, they're not actually high in calories – about 80 for a medium-sized egg. So a two-egg omelette with a non-fatty filling made with no added fat in a non-stick pan is a tasty low-calorie meal. A fresh herb omelette with a yoghurt and tarragon-vinegar dressed salad is a banquet! It's the overall amount of saturated fat which tends to push up the amount of cholesterol in our blood and the amount of cholesterol from egg yolks is fairly insignificant (provided you're not eating a dozen eggs a week, of course). Three eggs a week is a good balance to aim for.
- Most fruit and vegetables contain only minimal quantities of fat (until we try to improve on nature). One that contains a significant quantity is avocado. A pity because it's delicious. We don't need to stop eating them, but we should be aware that it's the one fruit or vegetable that's in the 'sometimes' category. Half an avocado with an oil-based vinaigrette is quite a fattening first course.

Where's the sugar?

Remember that, on average, we each eat about a hundred-weight of sugar a year: getting on for two pounds (just under a kilo) a week. So sugar is giving us a staggering 400-500 calories a day. About half of this sugar is under our direct control – we ourselves add it to our food. The other half is already present in a wide range of food we eat and so is less under our direct control – but with some knowledge and a little thought, we can reduce our sugar intake even from this area quite considerably.

Remember also that when cutting down on sugar, we're only cutting down on calories: we get virtually no other nutrients from sugar at all.

- Don't take sugar in tea or coffee. Even if you have a sweet tooth, you really can learn to enjoy tea and coffee without sugar. I know because I now couldn't drink either with sugar yet a few years ago I thought I couldn't drink coffee without sugar. This is a simple change to make to reduce your sugar consumption for life.

- You need to make your own mind up about swapping sugar for artificial sweeteners. If you have a craving for sweet things you need to master it so you only indulge occasionally: I don't think artificial sweeteners help you to do this. By the way, the artificial sweetener sorbitol, used in most diabetic sweets and chocolates, contains as many calories as sugar.
- Cut out fizzy canned drinks which are high in sugar – ten teaspoonsful a can. Either switch to low-cal drinks or, better, drink sparkling mineral water with ice and lemon, or unsweetened fruit juices.
- Cut out sweet snacks, biscuits, chocolates, cakes – choose fresh fruit instead where, remember, the sugar is well wrapped up in lots of fibre.
- Use tinned fruit packed in natural fruit juice rather than packed in sugar syrup – it's actually much more pleasant, and now very easily available in shops.
- Don't add sugar to your breakfast cereal – and first check that the manufacturer hasn't been there before you. Many breakfast cereals, including some which are promoted as 'healthy', have significant added sugar, and sometimes salt as well. Read the ingredients and make sure there is no added sugar.
- Read the label before you consume anything from a packet or can. You may still want to choose some of this food, but it's as well to know that the calorie count may be higher than you think.
- If you are buying processed food look for labels proclaiming 'reduced sugar' or 'no added sugar'. So many things now – from baked beans to jams – offer a 'reduced sugar' choice and it's wise to take it. You may be surprised to discover, by the way, how many things sugar is added to – from soups and sauces to pickles and peas.
- Even reduced-sugar jams contain significant calories, so go sparingly with them or, even better, save them for an occasional treat when you've reached your ideal weight.
- When you're making cakes, pies and other sweet things for the family (but not for you until you've lost weight!) try gradually cutting down the sugar you add. Aim over a few weeks to cut it by half. If there are complaints (which with

most things there probably won't be) increase the sugar a little next time. You should be able to get approval and still reduce the sugar content of your family's diet – sneaky eh?

Where's the fibre?

At last something you can eat more of! Here's a list of fibre-rich foods followed by some suggestions of the amounts you should be eating in your BBC Diet. Remember too that, for your health's sake, you should be eating at least this amount of fibre for life.

Fibre-rich foods include:
Wholemeal bread
Wholemeal flour
Brown rice
Wholemeal pasta
Wholemeal breakfast cereals
Bulgar or burghul wheat
Other grains like millet and buckwheat
Lentils
Peas – all kinds from split to frozen
Beans – all kinds from baked to cannelini
Chick peas
Sweetcorn
Potatoes – baked in the jacket
 or boiled in the skin
Green leafy vegetables, like spinach
Dried fruits

- Try to start the day with muesli or a wholemeal breakfast cereal with no added sugar.
- Eat two slices of wholemeal bread a day when you're losing weight; four slices if you can when you're at your ideal weight. Remember that bread helps to fill you without fattening you. If you need to spread it with something, use a thin smear of low-fat spread. Make sure you get 'wholemeal' rather than just 'brown' or 'wheatmeal' as these contain less fibre. White bread, by the way, isn't 'bad', it's just that it contains only a quarter of the fibre of wholemeal.
- With your main meal try to have a helping of one of the following:
    Potatoes (4-8 oz, 100-200 g), scrubbed not peeled, either baked or boiled
    Brown rice (2-3 oz, 50-75 g)

Wholewheat pasta (2-3 oz, 50-75 g)
Bulgar wheat (2-3 oz, 50-75 g)

The smaller amount is for when you want to lose weight as quickly as possible; the larger for when you've lost it or if you're content to lose it a little more slowly.

- Try to eat a portion of peas or beans or other pulses once a day.
- Eat at least one other portion of fresh vegetables a day. All vegetables contain some fibre, but the really fibre-rich ones are listed above. Salad vegetables like lettuce, tomatoes, cucumbers and celery don't contain very much fibre, but you can eat them freely as they also don't contain many calories.
- Eat two or three pieces of fresh fruit every day. Again, all fruit contains some fibre, though it's not particularly rich in it. It will help to fill you up, though, without providing too many calories. Dried fruit is higher in fibre but is also higher in calories so don't nibble too much 'neat'. Once you've soaked and cooked it, it contains much more water, so, weight for weight, contains fewer calories.

Where else can we cut calories?

In one word: alcohol. The average person will be taking perhaps 10 per cent of their daily calorie consumption from alcohol. This is drinking perhaps two or three drinks a day. You can cut these 200-300 calories at a stroke. Whether you want to or not is another matter. You may decide you'd rather lose weight a little more slowly and continue to drink moderately. It's important to remember that alcohol is 'empty' calories – supplying us with no nutrients. So don't substitute alcohol for food; if you want to try to lose weight on 1000 calories a day, you must add your calories from alcohol on top of this and accept that your weight loss will be slightly less rapid.

Very roughly – and as accurately as you need to know – one glass of wine and half a pint of beer and one single (pub measure) of spirits with a mixer are about 100 calories each. You should stick to only one measure of one of them a day if you want to lose weight.

Also, each of those measures contains one unit of alcohol. For your health's sake,

- men should not drink more than 21 units of alcohol a week – that's three a day

- women should not drink more than 14 units of alcohol a week – that's two a day

  Again, in this instance, safeguarding your health will also safeguard your figure.

DO I TAKE MY OWN MEDICINE?

A couple of years ago, I produced a television series and wrote a book called *Don't Break Your Heart* about how to avoid a heart attack. The evidence is impressive that the individual can reduce his or her risk of a heart attack and I changed my lifestyle then – changed my diet, lost weight, and started exercising regularly. Since then, I have to admit, although most of the healthy eating habits are still there, a few of the unhealthy ones have crept back too. And so, over the past year, my weight has increased again. I'm 5′ 9″ (1 m 72 cm) so my ideal weight is 12 stone (87 kg) or under. Just before starting writing this book, my weight had crept up to 13 st 12 lb (just under 100 kg). (It was just after Christmas!) I wanted to lose weight anyway as I was beginning to feel uncomfortable, but writing this book was an additional spur. I began to follow the guidelines which appear above.

First week I tried them but was somewhat thwarted as I had to eat out several times. I lost 4 lb (1.75 kg) this week.

Second week I'd started writing this book but I stuck to the guidelines reasonably well (though not, as you'll see, completely). I lost a further 6 lb (2.75 kg).

Third week I followed the guidelines rather less vigorously – with a little chocolate here and there! I lost a further 2 lb (1 kg).

Fourth week. This saw even more chocolate consumed (I was having to meet the deadline for the book). The rest of the time I did stick to the guidelines though and I lost a further 2 lb (1 kg).

So, over the month I lost 1 stone (7.25 kg) – I can honestly say fairly easily. Of course, I had several advantages:

- I'm male, which means it's easier for me to lose weight on more calories than a woman.

- This was the beginning of a diet, which is of course the time it's easiest to lose weight.

- I was taking regular exercise, a half hour's squash four or five times a week. (All the rest of the time, I was sitting writing or in bed!)

I know that without feeling deprived, I can continue to lose weight at the rate of 2 lb (1 kg) a week so should be at my ideal weight in another two months.

I thought it would be useful to share with you what I ate in the week I lost the most weight – 6 lb (2.75 kg). This will give you an idea of how I followed the guidelines and also where I cheated – I could have done better, but then I'm not perfect!

Day One **Wednesday** **Weight 13 st 8 lb** (94 kg)

Breakfast 1 white coffee (I was using semi-skimmed milk in tea and coffee. No sugar).
Mid-morning 1 white coffee; 1 satsuma; 2 shortbread biscuits.
Lunch 1 sardine, lettuce, cucumber and tomato sandwich (all the time during this week for sandwiches I used two slices of wholemeal bread – thinly spread with low-fat spread); 1 glass of unsweetened orange juice; 1 white coffee.
Mid-afternoon 1 cup of tea.
Dinner 3 oz (75 g) Rigatoni; sauce made with 15 oz (425 g) can tomatoes and 8 oz (200 g) of leftover roast lamb; onion, garlic, red pepper (this made three portions – I ate one now and froze two); 1 glass red wine; 1 pear; 1 white coffee.

- I made the classic error today of not eating breakfast. I needed 2 shortbread biscuits (after trying a satsuma) later in the morning
- I could have had 100 fewer calories by not having wine
- The Rigatoni was white pasta – I should get to like wholewheat pasta. I've done it with rice – I used to prefer white rice but now I prefer, by far, brown rice.

Day Two **Thursday**

Breakfast 1 white coffee; 1 slice wholemeal bread and low-fat spread and apricot jam.
Lunch 1 cheese and tomato pickle sandwich (cheese = 'low fat' cheddar type); 1 glass of orange juice, fresh, unsweetened; 1

mouthful of a custard slice (I wouldn't have been tempted had someone not been eating the rest!); 1 white coffee.

Mid-afternoon 1 cup of tea.

Dinner 3 oz (75g) noodles, uncooked weight (again wholewheat); 6 oz (150 g) haddock cooked in microwave in greaseproof paper envelope with ginger, garlic, spring onions, 1 tsp soy sauce and 2 tbsp dry vermouth; 4 oz (100 g) Chinese leaves microwaved in 2 tbsp oyster sauce; 1 glass red wine; 1 white coffee.

Day Three   Friday

Breakfast 1 white coffee; 1 slice of wholemeal bread with low-fat spread and apricot jam.

Mid-morning An apple.

Lunch 1 tuna, tomato and cucumber sandwich with 1 tsp low-fat fromage-frais and lemon juice; 1 glass orange juice; 1 white coffee.

Mid-afternoon 1 cup of tea.

Dinner tuna risotto with 1 tbsp olive oil, onion, garlic, $\frac{1}{3}$ can tuna in brine, 3 oz (75 g) brown rice, uncooked weight, 2 oz (50 g) frozen peas; radicchio, watercress and cucumber salad with dressing made from 1 tsp olive oil; 1 glass red wine; 1 white coffee.

- Again, tuna risotto was filling (I don't mind tuna twice in a day – but remember it's not compulsory!)
- I could have saved about 120 calories by not having 1 tbsp olive oil in the salad dressing; I could have used low-fat yoghurt dressing instead.

Day Four   Saturday

Breakfast 1 white coffee; 2 Weetabix with $\frac{1}{2}$ oz (15 g) sugar and semi-skimmed milk (I can't eat them without sugar – yet!).

Lunch 1 pack of Tesco's vegetable chilli with some of a white baguette; 1 glass orange juice; 1 apple; 1 white coffee.

Mid-afternoon 1 cup of tea; clementine; 1 handful grapes.

Dinner 3 oz (75 g) *wholewheat* noodles, uncooked weight (I was forcing myself, I still prefer white); beef and red pepper in blackbean sauce (made with 5 oz (125 g) thinly sliced lean steak); 1 330 ml can of lager; 2 oz (50 g) apricots; 2 tbsp low-fat natural yoghurt (dried apricots cooked in just enough water to cover – no sugar); 1 black coffee.

- Chinese noodles – both white and wholewheat take only four minutes to cook; about the same length of time it took to stir-fry the beef in blackbean sauce (using 2 tsp of sesame oil).

Day Five   Sunday

Breakfast 1 white coffee; unsweetened muesli with semi-skimmed milk.

Lunch Pre-lunch drink of sparkling mineral water with a couple of drops of angostura bitters, ice and lemon! (You can see here I was trying.); raw carrot fingers to nibble; roast chicken breast, without skin, steamed whole potatoes, leeks, carrots, broad beans, thickened gravy (most of the fat spooned off); 1 glass of red wine; apricot fool – made with cooked dried apricots, low-fat fromage-frais, low-fat natural yoghurt; 1 white coffee.

Mid-afternoon 1 cup of tea.

Supper 1 chicken and watercress sandwich; 1 glass of orange juice; 2 clementines; handful of grapes; 1 white coffee.

- Remember you halve the fat by taking the skin off the roast chicken – painful for me as I love it, but I did it. Fortunately, it loses its appeal when it's cold.
- Spooning all the fat off and not thickening the gravy results in fewer calories.

Day Six   Monday

Breakfast 1 white coffee; muesli with semi-skimmed milk and apricots (dried apricots cooked go a long way! – and keep for days in the fridge).

Lunch 1 chicken sandwich with tomato and cucumber; 1 glass of orange juice; 1 banana; 1 white coffee.

Mid-afternoon 1 cup of tea.

Supper 2 slices wholemeal toast with 16 oz (450 g) can of baked beans (reduced-sugar baked beans).

- This was not the supper I'd intended. I had to go out for a few hours for a meeting and returned to find my house had been burgled! Amongst other things taken was my microwave oven with the half-eaten chicken of the day before! I did feel like turning to a big Chinese take-away for comfort but decided on baked beans on toast instead. (This is a lot of baked beans on toast: one could manage on half the quantity.)

Day Seven   Tuesday

Breakfast 1 white coffee; unsweetened muesli with semi-skimmed milk.

Lunch 1 ham sandwich (2 oz (50 g), fat cut off) with tomato and cucumber; 1 glass orange; 1 white coffee.

Mid-afternoon 1 cup of tea.

Dinner Sardines (fresh i.e. frozen and thawed) stuffed with wholemeal breadcrumbs, garlic, lemon juice, parsley and sorrel (baked in foil in the oven), 1 baked potato with ¼ tsp low-fat spread; radicchio and watercress salad with low-fat yoghurt with tarragon vinegar dressing; 1 glass of red wine; handful of grapes; 1 white coffee (I avoided calories here by having an oil-free salad dressing).

Weight 13 st 2 lbs (91.25 kg) – a loss of 6 lb (2.75 kg) in the week.

As you can see, I followed the guidelines reasonably but not perfectly! I was aware when I was deviating so that I didn't stray too much. I actually weighed all the food I had (not the radicchio and watercress) and calculated the calories (just to prove that you don't need to!). Roughly, I had about 1500 calories a day. By having smaller portions (3 oz (75 g) brown rice, uncooked weight, is quite a lot!), cutting down oil more and not drinking alcohol, my calorie intake would have been nearer 1000 and I would have lost even more weight.

You may think my diet was a little monotonous, but it does show that you really don't need to starve or chew on lettuce leaves in order to lose weight – I never felt hungry – except before meals of course! I ate food which was quick to prepare as I was writing this book at the same time. And that's the other interesting thing. Writing a book (with a tight deadline) is quite stressful and when I'm stressed, I usually eat more 'for comfort', usually things like chocolate and biscuits. I proved to myself I didn't need to. (As I've already admitted though, when things became even more tense as the deadline approached, a bit of chocolate did sneak in – not too much though, and not sufficient to stop me continuing to lose weight.)

Now, if you don't fancy my week's version of the BBC Diet, here is a range of eating plans that you could follow.

THE DIET PLANS

If you prefer to have something more definite than guidelines, here is a range of BBC Diet plans, each for two weeks. As I've already said, you can follow them exactly or, if you prefer, use them as a basis for constructing your own plan. If you do deviate from the set plans, ensure that you are following the guidelines on fat, sugar and fibre. There are three basic plans:*

A *The short sharp shock!* This plan provides on average about 1000 calories a day. Anyone can use this plan for the most rapid results. But men and women who are average height or above and who are reasonably active, will achieve very satisfactory weight loss on the other plans. Women who are below average height and are inactive, may find that they only get a satisfactory weight loss if they stick to this plan. But if they do stick to this plan, *everyone* will lose weight. 1000 calories a day is the lowest number you should aim for in a diet lasting for a couple of weeks or more.

B *The middle way* This plan provides about 1250 calories a day and is the best plan for most women and for men who want to lose weight quickly.

C *Slower but sure* Most men will find that they lose at a satisfactory rate on this plan; and, of course, it's easier than the others as you're allowed to eat more: it provides about 1500 calories a day. In fact, most women who increase their physical activity will also lose weight on this plan at a slightly slower but still worthwhile rate.

> * Another way of using the plans is to alternate them: you could have two weeks on A, followed by two weeks on B, followed by two weeks on C. Or you could alternate between A and B or between B and C. Alternating may actually be more effective for you as you may find it easier to continue to diet, after the quick initial weight loss, by having easier and slightly 'harder' fortnights.

There are two other plans derived from our guidelines:

D *The easy way* This is my own ideal two-week plan. It's a 'middle way' diet and the vast majority of people will lose weight satisfactorily – and happily on it. When I look at it, I think I could stay on it for a lifetime – but as you've already seen, I do cheat a little: a little wine here, a little more oil there. This doesn't matter – it just means weight loss is a little less fast than it would otherwise be.

E *The gourmet plan* This is based on Anton Mosimann's recipes. This really is the Rolls Royce of slimming diets. If you're working all day, it would take quite a bit of organisation to follow it completely. One good way of following it would be when you're on holiday – it would be like having a luxury health farm holiday in your own home. Alternatively, you could incorporate it into another plan at weekends, or use it when you can follow the guidelines.

How to follow each of the plans

- First of all, each of the plans is quite flexible. You can interchange any of the days or meals. Remember though that the variety of food is important for a nutritious diet. Choose one breakfast from the lists, at the beginning of each diet plan, one snack meal and one main meal for each day.

- Try not to skip breakfast. If you eat then, it really will help you from being tempted to snack later. Of course, this isn't a rigid rule; you could eat what you should eat for breakfast as a snack later in the day.

- Allow yourself half-a-pint (300 ml) of skimmed milk a day. You'll find this is enough for your breakfast and for cups of coffee and tea throughout the day. There's no restriction on coffee or tea but don't add any sugar to them. If you need to, use artificial sweeteners.

- Don't drink any sweetened drinks. Try low-cal commercial drinks or drink unsweetened natural fruit juice (but not more than ⅓ pint (200 ml) a day). Drink plenty of water – this is important when you increase your fibre intake but it will also help to fill you up. It's a good idea always to have a glass of iced mineral water or plain tap water with each meal.

- If you want to lose weight quickly it's best to avoid alcohol. If you do want to drink alcohol, don't cut down on the food you're eating. Remember that alcohol only contains calories and no nutrients. So if you do drink, remember that you're adding calories and are slowing down your weight loss. Try to restrict yourself to a glass of wine or half a pint of beer – about 100 calories each day.

- As all these plans are based on healthy, as well as slimming, eating, it's quite safe to continue on one until you have reached your ideal weight.

Coping with temptation One of the advantages of the BBC Diet is that you shouldn't have to cope with too much temptation: you don't need to be on starvation rations and you don't need to feel hungry. Even when we're not hungry, though, we may be tempted by a biscuit or a piece of chocolate, which in turn tempts us to another. If you know you have weaknesses in this direction think out in advance ways of coping with them. Here are some effective ones:

- Remember you're not going to buy food which is fatty and sugary and is going to tempt you. If you have to buy it for the family, lock it away or get them to hide it. Write someone else's name on it.

- Make sure you have plenty of tempting non-fatty, non-sugary snack food around. Fresh fruit is your great friend. Buy plenty of it. Carry an apple or another fruit around with you. If you feel an urge to demolish a box of chocolates, promise yourself that you'll eat an apple – or preferably two – first. Then you'll be surprised at your strength in being able to overcome temptation.

- Always have in the fridge sticks of carrot, cucumber, celery, peppers or radishes or florets of cauliflower. Prepare them and keep them in a bowl of water or a polythene bag. Eat them when you're tempted by crisps or other savoury nibbles.

- Look at your food diary and see the times you're vulnerable and the food that tempts you. Work out how you'll cope with this. For example, if you know you just must have a couple of biscuits when you have a cup of tea – have a low-cal soft drink, or sparkling water and an apple instead.

- Don't eat when you're doing something else like reading or watching TV. When you eat, concentrate on the food and nothing else. Try to slow down your eating by savouring every mouthful. After you start eating, it takes twenty minutes or so for your stomach to signal 'full' to your appetite control centre in the brain. Give it a chance to work!

- Try only to eat at mealtimes. If you need to eat between meals, make it a healthy snack as outlined above, but before you eat anything, think, 'Can I do something else instead?' 'Can I do some gardening, call a friend, brush my teeth, take a shower, do some housework?!'

- Remember there are no forbidden foods, just food that you control your intake of. The idea is that you are in control. Don't drool over or become obsessed by foods. If you become fixated by a box of chocolates, eat your two apples and have one. If you resist and resist, you'll end up eating the whole box.

- In times of temptation look at your ten reasons for losing weight. Remember your contract and reward. Remember how many pounds you've lost: you've made an investment, don't start frittering it away.

DIET PLAN A: THE SHORT SHARP SHOCK!

For a flexible plan, choose one breakfast, one snack and one main meal per day.

Breakfasts

For one person:

1. 1 oz (25 g) branflakes
   ¼ pt (150 ml) skimmed milk
   1 slice wholemeal toast
   low fat spread

2. ¼ pt (150 ml) orange juice
   1 Weetabix
   ¼ pt (150 ml) skimmed milk

3. ¼ pt (150 ml) orange juice
   5 oz (125 g) porridge (oats and
     water)
   2 oz (50 g) chopped banana

4. 4 oz (100 g) grapefruit segments
   1 slice wholemeal toast
   low fat spread

5. 4 oz (100 g) grapefruit segments
   2 oz (50 g) prunes
   1 slice wholemeal toast
   low fat spread

6. 1 slice lean back bacon, grilled
   4 oz (100 g) tinned tomatoes
   1 slice wholemeal toast
   low fat spread

7. ¼ pt (150 ml) orange juice
   1 boiled egg
   1 slice wholemeal toast
   low fat spread

8. ¼ pt (150 ml) apple juice
   1½ oz (40 g) unsweetened muesli
   ¼ pt (150 ml) skimmed milk

9. 5 oz (150 g) porridge (oats and
     water)
   2 oz (50 g) chopped banana
   1 slice wholemeal toast
   low fat spread

10. ¼ pt (150 ml) orange juice
    1 slice wholemeal toast
    low fat spread

11. 1 Shredded Wheat
    ¼ pt (150 ml) skimmed milk
    2 oz (50 g) chopped banana

12. ¼ pt (150 ml) orange juice
    1 egg, scrambled with 2 fl oz
      (50 ml) skimmed milk in ⅛ oz
      (5 g) sunflower margarine
    1 slice wholemeal toast
    low fat spread

Snack meals

For one person:

1. ½ pt (150 ml) garden vegetable
     soup (p. 105)
   2 cream crackers
   2 oz (50 g) Edam or Brie cheese
   1 small banana or peach

2. 2 slices wholemeal bread
   2 oz (50 g) lean roast beef
   crunchy lettuce
   1 pear or 4 oz (100 g) strawberries

3. 5-7 oz (150-200 g) jacket potato
   4 oz (100 g) cottage cheese filling
   1 orange or 2 tangerines

4. 2 oz (50 g) corned beef
   2 slices wholemeal bread
   crunchy lettuce
   1 pear or 4 oz (100 g) cherries

5. 1 tuna pot rice (eat hot or cold)
     (p. 109)
   1 diet yoghurt

6. 4 oz (100 g) carton cottage
     cheese
   2 rye crispbreads
   2 small tomatoes
   1 diet yoghurt

7. 2 slices wholemeal bread
   2 oz (50 g) lean ham
   1 small tomato
   1 small banana or 4 oz (100 g)
     grapes

8. leek and carrot soup (p. 105)
   1 hard-boiled egg
   2 rye crispbreads
   crunchy lettuce
   1 apple or 1 slice fresh pineapple

9. 5-7 oz (150-200 g) jacket potato
   2 oz (50 g) chopped ham
   2 oz (50 g) mushrooms poached
     in skimmed milk
   1 diet yoghurt with 4 oz (100 g)
     chopped pear or whole
     strawberries

10. 2 slices wholemeal bread
    2 oz (50 g) Edam or Camembert
      cheese
    1 small tomato
    1 large orange or 4 oz (100 g)
      raspberries

11. 4 oz (100 g) carton cottage
      cheese
    4 oz (100 g) celery
      'strips to dip'
    2 oz (50 g) carrots
      'strips to dip'
    2 rye crispbreads
    1 apple or peach

12. 1 slice wholemeal bread
    2 oz (50 g) roast chicken
    1 medium tomato
    1 small banana or 4 oz (100 g)
      grapes

13. 5-7 oz (150-200 g) jacket potato
    2 small low-fat sausages, grilled
    4 oz (100 g) tinned tomatoes
    1 pear or 3 plums

14. 2 slices wholemeal bread
    2 oz (50 g) mashed sardines
    cucumber
    1 diet yoghurt

Main meals

For one person:

1. fisherman's pie (p. 108)
   2 oz (50 g) peas or broccoli
   2 oz (50 g) carrots or courgettes
   1 slice wholemeal bread
   low fat spread
   1 diet yoghurt

2. beef casserole (p. 115)
   2 oz (50 g) green beans
   1 apple or 4 oz (100 g) cherries

3. tuna pasta ribbons (p. 113)
   1 diet yoghurt with 4 oz (100 g)
      chopped apple

4. pork and pineapple (p. 108)
   4 oz (100 g) brown rice,
      cooked weight
   green salad (without dressing)
   spicy pear and orange (p. 116)

5. grilled chicken rosemary (p. 110)
   5-7 oz (150-200 g) jacket potato
   2 oz (50 g) sliced green beans
   4 oz (100 g) fresh fruit salad

6. Spanish omelette (p. 106)
   2 oz (50 g) mushrooms poached
      in skimmed milk
   1 slice wholemeal bread
   low fat spread
   baked banana and orange (p. 115)

7. 4 oz (100 g) lean roast leg of
      lamb
   5-7 oz (150-200 g) jacket potato
   2 oz (50 g) peas or cauliflower
   2 oz (50 g) swede or spinach
   chopped apple crunch (p. 116)

8. chilli mince (p. 114)
   small crusty roll
   green salad (without dressing)
   4 oz (100 g) fresh fruit salad

9. crunchy fish bake (p. 112)
   4 oz (100 g) baked tomatoes
   2 oz (50 g) peas or leeks
   baked banana and orange (p. 115)

10. soufflé herb omelette (p. 106)
    5-7 oz (150-200 g) jacket potato
    2 oz (50 g) green beans or
       courgettes
    1 diet yoghurt

11. chicken curry (p. 111)
    4 oz (100 g) brown rice,
       cooked weight
    green salad (without dressing)
    4 oz (100 g) stewed pear
    2 oz (50 g) vanilla ice-cream

12. vegetable and bean hot pot
       (p. 112)
    small crunchy roll
    1 diet yoghurt

13. macaroni cottage cheese (p. 107)
    green salad (without dressing)
    1 slice wholemeal toast
    fresh fruit salad

14. 4 oz (100 g) roast chicken, skin
       removed
    5-7 oz (150-200 g) jacket potato
    2 oz (50 g) peas
    2 oz (50 g) carrots or leeks
    spicy pear and orange (p. 116)

DIET PLAN A: THE SHORT SHARP SHOCK!

Day 1
1 oz (25 g) branflakes
¼ pt (150 ml) skimmed milk
1 slice wholemeal toast
low fat spread

¼ pt (150 ml) garden vegetable
    soup (p. 105)
2 cream crackers
2 oz (50 g) Edam or Brie cheese
1 small banana or peach

fisherman's pie (p. 108)
2 oz (50 g) carrots or broccoli
2 oz (50 g) peas or courgettes
1 slice wholemeal bread
low fat spread
1 diet yoghurt

¼ pt (150 ml) skimmed milk for
    drinks

Day 2
¼ pt (150 ml) orange juice
1 Weetabix
¼ pt (150 ml) skimmed milk

2 slices wholemeal bread
2 oz (50 g) lean roast beef
crunchy lettuce
1 pear or 4 oz (100 g) strawberries

beef casserole (p. 115)
2 oz (50 g) green beans
1 apple or 4 oz (100 g) cherries

¼ pt (150 ml) skimmed milk for
    drinks

Day 3
¼ pt (150 ml) orange juice
5 oz (125 g) porridge
2 oz (50 g) chopped banana

5-7 oz (150-200 g) jacket potato
4 oz (100 g) cottage cheese filling
1 orange or 2 tangerines

tuna pasta ribbons (p. 113)
1 diet yoghurt with 4 oz (100 g)
    chopped apple

¼ pt (150 ml) skimmed milk for
    drinks

Day 4
4 oz (100 g) grapefruit segments
2 slices wholemeal toast
low fat spread

2 oz (50 g) corned beef
2 slices wholemeal bread
crunchy lettuce
1 pear or 4 oz (100 g) cherries

pork and pineapple (p. 108)
4 oz (100 g) brown rice, cooked
    weight
green salad (without dressing)
spicy pear and orange (p. 116)

¼ pt (150 ml) skimmed milk for
    drinks

Day 5

4 oz (100 g) unsweetened
  grapefruit segments
2 oz (50 g) unsweetened prunes
1 slice wholemeal toast
low fat spread

tuna pot rice (p. 109)
1 diet yoghurt

grilled chicken rosemary (p. 110)
5-7 oz (150-200 g) jacket potato
2 oz (50 g) sliced green beans
4 oz (100 g) fresh fruit salad

¼ pt (150 ml) skimmed milk for
  drinks

Day 6

1 slice lean back bacon, grilled
4 oz (100 g) tinned tomatoes
1 slice wholemeal toast
low fat spread

4 oz (100 g) carton cottage cheese
2 rye crispbread
2 small tomatoes
1 diet yoghurt

Spanish omelette (p. 106)
2 oz (50 g) mushrooms poached in
  skimmed milk
1 slice wholemeal bread
low fat spread
baked banana and orange (p. 115)

¼ pt (150 ml) skimmed milk for
  drinks

Day 7

¼ pt (150 ml) orange juice
1 boiled egg
1 slice wholemeal toast
low fat spread

2 slices wholemeal bread
2 oz (50 g) lean ham
1 small tomato
1 small banana or 4 oz (100 g)
  grapes

4 oz (100 g) lean roast leg of lamb
5-7 oz (150-200 g) jacket potato
2 oz (50 g) peas or cauliflower
2 oz (50 g) swede or spinach
chopped apple crunch (p. 116)

¼ pt (150 ml) skimmed milk for
  drinks

Day 8

¼ pt (150 ml) apple juice
1½ oz (40 g) unsweetened muesli
¼ pt (150 ml) skimmed milk

leek and carrot soup (p. 105)
1 hard-boiled egg
2 rye crispbreads
crunchy lettuce
1 apple or 1 slice fresh pineapple

chilli mince (p. 114)
small crusty roll
green salad (without dressing)
4 oz (100 g) fresh fruit salad

¼ pt (150 ml) skimmed milk for
  drinks

Day 9
¼ pt (150 ml) orange juice
1 Weetabix
¼ pt (150 ml) skimmed milk

5-7 oz (150-200 g) jacket potato
2 oz (50 g) chopped ham
2 oz (50 g) mushrooms poached in
  skimmed milk
1 diet yoghurt with 4 oz (100 g)
  chopped pear or whole
  strawberries

crunchy fish bake (p. 112)
4 oz (100 g) baked tomatoes
2 oz (50 g) peas or leeks
baked banana and orange (p. 115)

¼ pt (150 ml) skimmed milk for
  drinks

Day 10
5 oz (150 g) porridge
  2 oz (50 g) chopped banana
1 slice wholemeal toast
low fat spread

2 slices wholemeal bread
2 oz (50 g) Edam or Camembert
  cheese
1 small tomato
1 large orange or 4 oz (100 g)
  raspberries

soufflé herb omelette (p. 106)
5-7 oz (150-200 g) jacket potato
2 oz (50 g) green beans or
  courgettes
1 diet yoghurt

¼ pt (150 ml) skimmed milk for
  drinks

Day 11
4 oz (100 g) grapefruit segments
2 oz (50 g) prunes
1 slice wholemeal toast
low fat spread

4 oz (100 g) carton cottage cheese
4 oz (100 g) celery
  'strips to dip'
2 oz (50 g) carrots
  'strips to dip'
2 rye crispbreads
1 apple or peach

chicken curry (p. 111)
4 oz (100 g) brown rice, cooked
  weight
green salad (without dressing)
4 oz (100 g) stewed pear
2 oz (50 g) vanilla ice-cream

¼ pt (150 ml) skimmed milk for
  drinks

Day 12
¼ pt (150 ml) orange juice
1 slice wholemeal toast
low fat spread

1 slice wholemeal bread
2 oz (50 g) liver pâté
1 medium tomato
1 small banana or 3 plums

vegetable and bean hot pot (p. 112)
small crunchy roll
1 diet yoghurt

¼ pt (150 ml) skimmed milk for
  drinks

Day 13

1 Shredded Wheat
¼ pt (150 ml) skimmed milk
2 oz (50 g) chopped banana

5-7 oz (150-200 g) jacket potato
2 small low-fat sausages, grilled
4 oz (100 g) tinned tomatoes
1 pear

macaroni cottage cheese (p. 107)
green salad (without dressing)
1 slice wholemeal toast
4 oz (100 g) fresh fruit salad

¼ pt (150 ml) skimmed milk for
drinks

Day 14

¼ pt (150 ml) orange juice
1 egg, scrambled with 2 fl oz (50
ml) skimmed milk in ⅛ oz (5 g)
sunflower margarine
1 slice wholemeal toast
low fat spread

2 slices wholemeal bread
2 oz (50 g) mashed sardines
cucumber
1 diet yoghurt

4 oz (100 g) roast chicken, with the
skin removed
5-7 oz (150-200 g) jacket potato
2 oz (50 g) peas
2 oz (50 g) carrots or leeks
spicy pear and orange (p. 116)

¼ pt (150 ml) skimmed milk for
drinks

DIET PLAN B:
THE MIDDLE WAY

For a flexible plan, choose one breakfast, one snack and one main meal per day.

Breakfasts

For one person:

1. ¼ pt (150 ml) orange juice
   2 Weetabix
   ¼ pt (150 ml) skimmed milk

2. 4 oz (100 g) unsweetened
   grapefruit segments
   2 slices wholemeal toast
   low fat spread

3. ¼ pt (150 ml) apple juice
   2 oz (50 g) unsweetened muesli
   ¼ pt (150 ml) skimmed milk

4. 1 oz (25 g) branflakes
   ¼ pt (150 ml) skimmed milk
   1 slice wholemeal toast
   low fat spread

5. ¼ pt (150 ml) orange juice
   6 oz (150 g) porridge
   2 oz (50 g) chopped banana
   1 slice wholemeal bread
   low fat spread

6. ¼ pt (150 ml) orange juice
   1 boiled egg
   1 slice wholemeal toast
   low fat spread

7. 1 Shredded Wheat
   ¼ pt (150 ml) skimmed milk
   1 slice wholemeal toast
   low fat spread

8. ¼ pt (150 ml) orange juice
   1 oz (25 g) branflakes
   ¼ pt (150 ml) skimmed milk
   2 oz (50 g) chopped banana

9. 4 oz (100 g) unsweetened
   grapefruit segments
   2 oz (50 g) unsweetened prunes
   2 slices wholemeal toast
   sunflower margarine

10. ¼ pt (150 ml) orange juice
    1 egg, scrambled with 2 fl oz (50
    ml) skimmed milk in ⅛ oz (5 g)
    sunflower margarine
    1 slice wholemeal toast
    low fat spread

11. 2 rashers lean back bacon, grilled
    5 oz (125 g) tinned tomatoes
    1 slice wholemeal toast
    low fat spread

Sandwich-based snacks

For one person:

1. 2 slices wholemeal bread
   2 oz (50 g) Edam or Brie cheese
   1 small tomato
   1 large orange or 4 oz (100 g
   grapes

2. 2 slices wholemeal bread
   2 oz (50 g) tuna
   1 oz (25 g) cucumber
   1 pear or 4 oz (100 g)
   strawberries

3. 2 slices wholemeal bread
   2 oz (50 g) cottage cheese
   ½ oz (15 g) cucumber
   1 small banana or 4 oz (100 g)
   raspberries

4. 2 slices wholemeal bread
   2 oz (50 g) corned beef
   crunchy lettuce
   1 orange or 2 tangerines

5. 2 slices wholemeal bread
   2 oz (50 g) mashed sardines
   cucumber and cress
   1 diet yoghurt

6. 2 slices wholemeal bread
   1 hard-boiled egg, finely chopped
   with onion and cress
   1 apple or 1 slice fresh pineapple

7. 2 slices wholemeal bread
   2 oz (50 g) roast chicken
   crunchy lettuce
   1 small tomato
   1 pear or 4 oz (100 g)
   strawberries

8. 2 slices wholemeal bread
   2 oz (50 g) low fat Cheddar
   ½ oz (15 g) finely chopped onion
   1 diet yoghurt

9. 2 slices wholemeal bread
   2 oz (50 g) lean ham
   1 small tomato
   1 small banana or 4 oz (100 g)
   grapes

10. 2 slices wholemeal bread
    2 oz (50 g) chicken
    1 small tomato
    1 apple or 3 plums

Snack meals

For one person:

1. tuna pot rice (p. 109)

2. 5 oz (125 g) baked beans
   2 slices wholemeal toast
   1 diet yoghurt

3. 4 oz (100 g) low-fat burger,
   grilled
   wholemeal bun

4. 7-9 oz (200-250 g) jacket potato
   2 small low-fat sausages, grilled

5. 7-9 oz (200-250 g) jacket potato
   3 oz (75 g) cottage cheese

6. 7-9 oz (200-250 g) jacket potato
   2 oz (50 g) Cheddar cheese
   1 oz (25 g) onion

7. 7-9 oz (200-250 g) jacket potato
   2 oz (50 g) chilli mince (p. 114)

8. 7-9 oz (200-250 g) jacket potato
   5 oz (150 g) baked beans

9. 7-9 oz (200-250 g) jacket potato
   2 oz (50 g) chopped ham
   2 oz (50 g) chopped mushrooms
       poached in skimmed milk

10. Spanish omelette (p. 106)
    1 slice wholemeal bread

11. scrambled eggs on toast (see
        breakfast menu – use 2 eggs
        and omit fruit juice)

Main meals

For one person:

1. 6 oz (150 g) gammon steak,
       grilled
   pineapple ring
   2 oz (50 g) sweetcorn or peas
   4 oz (100 g) baked tomato
   7-9 oz (200-250 g) baked potato
   baked banana and orange (p. 115)

2. chilli mince (p. 114)
   4 oz (100 g) brown rice, cooked
       weight
   4 oz (100 g) fresh fruit salad
   2 oz (50 g) ice-cream

3. Spanish omelette (p. 106)
   2 oz (50 g) mushrooms poached
       in skimmed milk
   5 oz (150 g) tinned tomatoes
   1 slice wholemeal bread
   low fat spread
   1 diet yoghurt

4. tuna pasta ribbons (p. 113)
   1 slice wholemeal bread
   chopped apple crunch (p. 116)

5. grilled chicken rosemary (p. 110)
   ratatouille (p. 107)
   4 oz (100 g) boiled, sliced potato
   spicy pear and orange (p. 116)

6. sardine and tomato pizza (p. 109)
   green salad
   7-9 oz (200-250 g) jacket potato
   1 apple or 4 oz (100 g)
       strawberries

7. 4 oz (100 g) roast chicken with
       skin removed
   7-9 oz (200-250 g) jacket potato
   2 oz (50 g) peas or courgettes
   2 oz (50 g) carrots or cabbage
   1 tablespoon stuffing and gravy
   baked apple and sultanas (p. 116)

8. 4 oz (100 g) lean lamb chop and
       rosemary, grilled
   8 oz (200 g) boiled potato with
       skin on
   4 oz (100 g) baked tomatoes
   2 oz (50 g) peas or leeks
   4 oz (100 g) chopped apple and
       1 diet yoghurt

9. beef and vegetable curry (p. 111)
   4 oz (100 g) brown rice, cooked
      weight
   wholemeal roll
   tomato and onion salad (made
      with 2 small tomatoes)
   2 oz (50 g) vanilla ice-cream

10. beef casserole (p. 115)
    7-9 oz (200-250 g) jacket potato
    2 oz (50 g) carrots or green beans
    chopped apple crunch (p. 116)

11. fisherman's pie (p. 108)
    2 oz (50 g) peas or broccoli
    2 oz (50 g) carrots or leeks
    wholemeal roll
    2 oz (50 g) sliced banana or
       strawberries and
       1 diet yoghurt

12. chicken and vegetable risotto
       (p. 111)
    wholemeal roll
    green salad (without dressing)
    fresh fruit salad

13. macaroni cottage cheese (p. 107)
    1 rasher lean back bacon, grilled
    1 slice wholemeal bread
    spicy pear and orange (p. 116)

14. 4 oz (100 g) lean roast lamb and
       mint sauce
    7-9 oz (200-250 g) jacket potato
    2 oz (50 g) cabbage or leeks
    2 oz (50 g) swede or green beans
    baked banana and orange
       (p. 115)

DIET PLAN B:
THE MIDDLE WAY

Day 1

¼ pt (150 ml) unsweetened orange
   juice
2 Weetabix
¼ pt (150 ml) skimmed milk

2 slices wholemeal bread
2 oz (50 g) mashed sardines
cucumber and cress
1 diet yoghurt

6 oz (150 g) grilled gammon steak
pineapple ring
2 oz (50 g) sweetcorn or peas
4 oz (100 g) baked tomato
7-9 oz (200-250 g) jacket potato
baked banana and orange (p. 115)

¼ pt (150 ml) skimmed milk for
   drinks

Day 2

4 oz (100 g) unsweetened
   grapefruit segments
2 slices wholemeal toast
low fat spread

4 oz (100 g) low-fat burger, grilled
wholemeal bun
1 apple

chilli mince (p. 114)
4 oz (100 g) brown rice, cooked
   weight
4 oz (100 g) fresh fruit salad
2 oz (50 g) vanilla ice-cream

¼ pt (150 ml) skimmed milk for
   drinks

Day 3

¼ pt (150 ml) apple juice
2 oz (50 g) unsweetened muesli
¼ pt (150 ml) skimmed milk

2 slices wholemeal bread
2 oz (50 g) roast chicken
crunchy lettuce
1 small tomato
1 pear or 4 oz (100 g) strawberries

Spanish omelette (p. 106)
2 oz (50 g) mushrooms poached in
   skimmed milk
5 oz (150 g) tinned tomatoes
1 slice wholemeal bread
low fat spread
1 diet yoghurt

¼ pt (150 ml) skimmed milk for
   drinks

Day 4

1 oz (25 g) branflakes
¼ pt (150 ml) skimmed milk
1 slice wholemeal toast
low fat spread

2 slices wholemeal bread
2 oz (50 g) low fat Cheddar or
   Edam
finely chopped onion
1 diet yoghurt

tuna pasta ribbons (p. 113)
1 slice wholemeal bread
chopped apple crunch (p. 116)

¼ pt (150 ml) skimmed milk for
   drinks

Day 5

¼ pt (150 ml) orange juice
6 oz (150 g) porridge
2 oz (50 g) chopped banana
1 slice wholemeal bread
low fat spread

tuna pot rice (p. 109)
1 diet yoghurt

grilled chicken rosemary (p. 110)
ratatouille (p. 107)
4 oz (100 g) boiled, sliced potato
spicy pear and orange (p. 116)

¼ pt (150 ml) skimmed milk for
    drinks

Day 6

2 rashers lean back bacon, grilled
5 oz (125 g) tinned tomatoes
1 slice wholemeal toast

5 oz (125 g) baked beans
2 slices wholemeal toast
1 diet yoghurt

sardine and tomato pizza (p. 109)
green salad (without dressing)
7-9 oz (200-250 g) jacket potato
1 apple or 4 oz (100 g) strawberries

¼ pt (150 ml) skimmed milk for
    drinks

Day 7

¼ pt (150 ml) orange juice
1 boiled egg
1 slice wholemeal toast
low fat spread

2 slices wholemeal bread
2 oz (50 g) lean ham
1 small tomato
1 small banana or 4 oz (100 g)
    grapes

4 oz (100 g) roast chicken, with
    skin removed
7-9 oz (200-250 g) jacket potato
2 oz (50 g) peas or courgettes
2 oz (50 g) carrots or cabbage
1 tablespoon stuffing and gravy
baked apple and sultanas (p. 116)

¼ pt (150 ml) skimmed milk for
    drinks

Day 8

1 Shredded Wheat
¼ pt (150 ml) skimmed milk
1 slice wholemeal toast
low fat spread

¼ pt (150 ml) garden vegetable
    soup (p. 105)
wholemeal roll
1 oz (25 g) low fat Cheddar or
    Edam
1 orange or tangerine

4 oz (100 g) lean lamb chop and
    rosemary, grilled
8 oz (200 g) boiled potato with skin
    on
4 oz (100 g) baked tomatoes
2 oz (50 g) peas or leeks
4 oz (100 g) chopped apple or
    strawberries and 1 diet yoghurt

¼ pt (150 ml) skimmed milk for
    drinks

Day 9

¼ pt (150 ml) orange juice
1 oz (25 g) branflakes
¼ pt (150 ml) skimmed milk
2 oz (50 g) chopped banana

7-9 oz (200-250 g) jacket potato
2 oz (50 g) tuna
1 oz (25 g) cucumber
1 pear

beef and vegetable curry (p. 111)
4 oz (100 g) brown rice, cooked
   weight
wholemeal roll
tomato and onion salad (made with
   2 small tomatoes)
2 oz (50 g) vanilla ice-cream

¼ pt (150 ml) skimmed milk for
   drinks

Day 10

4 oz (100 g) unsweetened
   grapefruit segments
2 oz (50 g) unsweetened prunes
2 slices wholemeal toast
low fat spread

2 slices wholemeal bread
½ oz (15 g) cucumber
2 oz (50 g) cottage cheese
1 small banana or 4 oz (100 g)
   raspberries

beef casserole (p. 115)
7-9 oz (200-250 g) jacket potato
2 oz (50 g) carrots or green beans
chopped apple crunch (p. 116)

¼ pt (150 ml) skimmed milk for
   drinks

Day 11

¼ pt (150 ml) orange juice
2 Weetabix
¼ pt (150 ml) skimmed milk

2 slices wholemeal bread
2 oz (50 g) lean roast beef
½ oz (15 g) crunchy lettuce
1 small tomato
1 pear

fisherman's pie (p. 108)
2 oz (50 g) carrots or broccoli
2 oz (50 g) peas or leeks
wholemeal roll
2 oz (50 g) sliced banana or
   strawberries and 1 diet yoghurt

¼ pt (150 ml) skimmed milk for
   drinks

Day 12

¼ pt (150 ml) orange juice
5 oz (150 g) porridge
2 oz (50 g) banana
1 slice wholemeal toast
low fat spread

2 slices wholemeal bread
2 oz (50 g) corned beef
½ oz (15 g) crunchy lettuce
1 orange

chicken and vegetable risotto
   (p. 111)
wholemeal roll
green salad (without dressing)
4 oz (100 g) fresh fruit salad

¼ pt (150 ml) skimmed milk for
   drinks

Day 13

¼ pt (150 ml) orange juice
1 egg scrambled with 2 fl oz (50 ml)
   skimmed milk in ⅛ oz (5 g)
   sunflower margarine
1 slice wholemeal toast
low fat spread

4 oz (100 g) low-fat burger, grilled
wholemeal bun
1 apple

macaroni cottage cheese (p. 107)
1 rasher lean back bacon, grilled
1 slice wholemeal toast
spicy pear and orange (p. 116)

¼ pt (150 ml) skimmed milk for
   drinks

Day 14

4 oz (100 g) unsweetened
   grapefruit segments
2 slices wholemeal toast
low fat spread

2 slices wholemeal bread
1 hard-boiled egg finely chopped
   with onion and cress
1 apple

4 oz (100 g) lean roast lamb and
   mint sauce
7-9 oz (200-250 g) jacket potato
2 oz (50 g) cabbage or leeks
2 oz (50 g) swede or green beans
baked banana and orange (p. 115)

¼ pt (150 ml) skimmed milk for
   drinks

DIET PLAN C: SLOWER BUT SURE

For a flexible plan, choose one breakfast, one snack and one main meal per day.

Breakfasts

For one person:

1. ¼ pt (150 ml) orange juice
   2 Weetabix
   ¼ pt (150 ml) skimmed milk
   1 slice wholemeal toast
   low fat spread

2. ¼ pt (150 ml) orange juice
   2 rashers lean back bacon, grilled
   2 slices wholemeal toast
   low fat spread

3. 2 rashers lean back bacon, grilled
   1 small low-fat sausage, grilled
   4 oz (100 g) tinned tomatoes
   1 slice wholemeal toast
   low fat spread

4. 2 eggs, scrambled with 2 fl oz
   (50 ml) skimmed milk in ¼ oz
   (10 g) sunflower margarine
   2 slices wholemeal toast
   low fat spread

5. ¼ pt (150 ml) orange juice
   5 oz (150 g) porridge
   4 oz (100 g) chopped banana
   2 slices wholemeal toast
   low fat spread

6. ¼ pt (150 ml) orange juice
   1 boiled egg
   2 slices wholemeal toast
   low fat spread

7. 1 oz (25 g) branflakes
   4 oz (100 g) chopped banana
   ¼ pt (150 ml) skimmed milk
   2 slices wholemeal toast
   low fat spread

8. ¼ pt (150 ml) orange juice
   1 Shredded Wheat
   ¼ pt (150 ml) skimmed milk
   2 slices wholemeal toast
   low fat spread

9. 2 rashers lean back bacon, grilled
   4 oz (100 g) tinned tomatoes
   2 oz (50 g) mushrooms
   1 slice wholemeal toast
   low fat spread

Sandwich-based snacks

For one person:

1. 3 slices wholemeal bread
   3 oz (75 g) Edam cheese
   1 medium tomato
   1 apple or 3 plums

2. 3 slices wholemeal bread
   smoked mackerel pâté (p. 110)
   cucumber
   1 apple or 4 oz (100 g) raspberries

3. 3 slices wholemeal bread
   2 oz (50 g) tuna
   lettuce
   1 small banana or 4 oz (100 g)
      fresh apricots

4. 3 slices wholemeal bread
   3 oz (75 g) lean ham
   1 medium tomato
   1 large orange or 1 slice fresh
      pineapple

5. 3 slices wholemeal bread
   3 oz (75 g) chicken breast, with
      skin removed
   cucumber
   1 pear or peach

6. 3 slices wholemeal bread
   3 oz (75 g) Edam or Brie cheese
   2 teaspoons Branston pickle
   1 apple or 4 oz (100 g)
      strawberries

7. 3 slices wholemeal bread
   3 oz (75 g) mashed sardines
   1 medium tomato
   1 apple

Main meals

For one person:

1. chunky vegetables and beef
      (p. 114)
   large crusty roll
   2 oz (50 g) peas or leeks
   spicy pear and orange (p. 116)
   4 oz (100 g) vanilla ice-cream

2. 4 oz (100 g) gammon, grilled
   7-9 oz (200-250 g) jacket potato
   2 oz (50 g) peas or leeks
   2 oz (50 g) sweetcorn
   4 oz (100 g) fresh fruit salad

3. chicken curry (p. 111)
   5 oz (150 g) brown rice, cooked
      weight
   tomato and onion salad (made
      with 2 small tomatoes)
   chopped apple crunch (p. 116)
   1 diet yoghurt

4. shepherd's pie (p. 114)
   4 oz (100 g) cauliflower or
      sprouts
   3 cream crackers
   2 oz (50 g) Edam or Brie cheese

5. chilli mince (p. 114)
   6 oz (150 g) brown rice, cooked
      weight
   green salad (without dressing)
   4 oz (100 g) fresh fruit salad
   4 oz (100 g) vanilla ice-cream

6. sardine and tomato pizza
      (p. 109)
   green salad (without dressing)
   9 oz (250 g) jacket potato
   2 cream crackers
   2 oz (50 g) Edam cheese

7. 4 oz (100 g) lean roast lamb
   9 oz (250 g) jacket potato
   2 oz (50 g) peas or spinach
   3 oz (75 g) cabbage or sprouts
   chopped apple crunch (p. 116)
   1 diet yoghurt

8. chicken and vegetable risotto
      (p. 111)
   2 oz (50 g) ice-cream

9. crunchy fish bake (p. 112)
   7-9 oz (200-250 g) jacket potato
   2 oz (50 g) carrots or courgettes
   baked banana and orange
      (p. 115)

10. beef and vegetable curry (p. 111)
    4 oz (100 g) brown rice, cooked
       weight
    2 oz (50 g) ice-cream
    4 oz (100 g) banana or 3 fresh
       apricots

11. pork and pineapple (p. 108)
    7-9 oz (200-250 g) baked potato
    4 oz (100 g) fresh fruit salad
    2 oz (50 g) ice-cream

12. tuna pasta ribbons (p. 113)
    1 slice wholemeal bread

13. liver with orange (p. 110)
    6 oz (150 g) brown rice, cooked
       weight
    2 oz (50 g) peas or leeks
    4 oz (100 g) ice-cream

14. 4 oz (100 g) roast chicken, skin
       removed
    8 oz (200 g) boiled potatoes
    2 oz (50 g) peas or courgettes
    2 oz (50 g) carrots or broccoli
    1 tablespoon stuffing and gravy
    baked apple and sultanas
       (p. 116)

DIET PLAN C:
SLOWER BUT SURE

Day 1

¼ pt (150 ml) orange juice
2 Weetabix
2 slices wholemeal toast
low fat spread
¼ pt (150 ml) skimmed milk

3 slices wholemeal bread
3 oz (75 g) lean ham
1 medium tomato
1 large orange or 1 slice fresh
  pineapple

chunky vegetables and beef
  (p. 114)
large crusty roll
2 oz (50 g) peas or leeks
spicy pear and orange (p. 116)
4 oz (100 g) vanilla ice-cream

¼ pt (150 ml) skimmed milk for
  drinks

Day 2

2 eggs scrambled with 2 fl oz (50
  ml) skimmed milk in ¼ oz (10 g)
  sunflower margarine
2 slices wholemeal toast
low fat spread

3 slices wholemeal bread
3 oz (75 g) Edam or Brie cheese
2 teaspoons Branston pickle
1 apple or 4 oz (100 g) strawberries

4 oz (100 g) gammon, grilled
7-9 oz (200-250 g) jacket potato
2 oz (50 g) peas or leeks
2 oz (50 g) sweetcorn
4 oz (100 g) fresh fruit salad

¼ pt (150 ml) skimmed milk for
  drinks

Day 3

1 oz (25 g) branflakes
4 oz (100 g) chopped banana
¼ pt (150 ml) skimmed milk
2 slices wholemeal toast
low fat spread

7-9 oz (200-250 g) jacket potato
5 oz (125 g) baked beans
1 orange

chicken curry (p. 111)
5 oz (125 g) brown rice, cooked
  weight
tomato and onion salad (made with
  2 small tomatoes)
chopped apple crunch (p. 116)
1 diet yoghurt

¼ pt (150 ml) skimmed milk for
  drinks

Day 4

¼ pt (150 ml) orange juice
5 oz (150 g) porridge
4 oz (100 g) chopped banana
2 slices wholemeal toast
low fat spread

3 slices wholemeal bread
smoked mackerel pâté (p. 110)
cucumber
1 apple or 4 oz (100 g) raspberries

shepherd's pie (p. 114)
4 oz (100 g) cauliflower or sprouts
3 cream crackers
2 oz (50 g) Edam or Brie cheese

¼ pt (150 ml) skimmed milk for
    drinks

Day 5

¼ pt (150 ml) orange juice
1 Shredded Wheat
¼ pt (150 ml) skimmed milk
2 slices wholemeal toast
low fat spread

3 slices wholemeal bread
3 oz (75 g) lean ham
1 medium tomato
1 large orange or 1 slice fresh
    pineapple

chilli mince (p. 114)
6 oz (150 g) brown rice, cooked
    weight
green salad (without dressing)
4 oz (100 g) fresh fruit salad
4 oz (100 g) vanilla ice-cream

¼ pt (150 ml) skimmed milk for
    drinks

Day 6

2 rashers lean back bacon, grilled
4 oz (100 g) tinned tomatoes
2 oz (50 g) mushrooms
2 slices wholemeal toast
low fat spread

3 slices wholemeal bread
3 oz (75 g) chicken breast with skin
    removed
cucumber
1 pear or peach

sardine and tomato pizza (p. 109)
green salad (without dressing)
9 oz (250 g) jacket potato
2 cream crackers
2 oz (50 g) Edam cheese

¼ pt (150 ml) skimmed milk for
    drinks

Day 7

1 oz (25 g) branflakes
4 oz (100 g) chopped banana
¼ pt (150 ml) skimmed milk
2 slices wholemeal toast
low fat spread

2-egg soufflé herb omelette (p. 106)
2 slices wholemeal bread
low fat spread
2 medium tomatoes
1 pear

4 oz (100 g) lean roast lamb
9 oz (250 g) jacket potato
2 oz (50 g) peas or spinach
3 oz (75 g) cabbage or sprouts
chopped apple crunch (p. 116)
1 diet yoghurt

¼ pt (150 ml) skimmed milk for
    drinks

Day 8

¼ pt (150 ml) orange juice
¼ pt (150 ml) skimmed milk
1 Shredded Wheat
2 slices wholemeal toast
low fat spread

3 slices wholemeal bread
2 oz (50 g) tuna
lettuce
1 small banana

chicken and vegetable risotto
    (p. 111)
2 oz (50 g) ice-cream
2 crackers
2 oz (50 g) Edam cheese

¼ pt (150 ml) skimmed milk for
    drinks

Day 9

¼ pt (150 ml) orange juice
2 slices wholemeal toast
2 oz (50 g) lean back bacon, grilled

9 oz (250 g) jacket potato
2 oz (50 g) Cheddar cheese
1 oz (25 g) onion, chopped
1 diet yoghurt

crunchy fish bake (p. 112)
8 oz (200 g) boiled/jacket potato
2 oz (50 g) carrots or courgettes
baked banana and orange (p. 115)
2 slices wholemeal toast
low fat spread

¼ pt (150 ml) skimmed milk for
    drinks

Day 10

¼ pt (150 ml) orange juice
2 Weetabix
¼ pt (150 ml) skimmed milk
2 slices wholemeal toast
low fat spread

3 slices wholemeal bread
3 oz (75 g) lean ham
1 medium tomato
1 orange

beef and vegetable curry (p. 111)
4 oz (100 g) brown rice, cooked
    weight
2 oz (50 g) ice-cream
4 oz (100 g) banana or 3 fresh
    apricots
2 crackers
2 oz (50 g) Edam cheese

¼ pt (150 ml) skimmed milk for
    drinks

Day 11

¼ pt (150 ml) orange juice
5 oz (150 g) porridge
4 oz (100 g) chopped banana
2 slices wholemeal toast
low fat spread

3 slices wholemeal bread
3 oz (75 g) mashed sardines
1 medium tomato
1 pear

pork and pineapple (p. 108)
8 oz (200 g) baked potato
4 oz (100 g) fresh fruit salad
2 oz (50 g) ice-cream

¼ pt (150 ml) skimmed milk for
    drinks

Day 12

¼ pt (150 ml) orange juice
1 Shredded Wheat
¼ pt (150 ml) skimmed milk
2 slices wholemeal toast
low fat spread

3 slices wholemeal bread
3 oz (75 g) Edam cheese
1 medium tomato
1 apple

tuna pasta ribbons (p. 113)
1 slice wholemeal bread
1 diet yoghurt

¼ pt (150 ml) skimmed milk for
    drinks

Day 13

2 rashers lean back bacon, grilled
1 small low-fat sausage, grilled
4 oz (100 g) tinned tomatoes
1 slice wholemeal toast
low fat spread

mushroom omelette (p. 106)
2 slices wholemeal bread
low fat spread
2 medium tomatoes
1 pear

liver with orange (p. 110)
6 oz (150 g) brown rice, cooked
    weight
2 oz (50 g) peas or leeks
4 oz (100 g) ice-cream

¼ pt (150 ml) skimmed milk for
    drinks

Day 14

1 oz (25 g) branflakes
¼ pt (150 ml) skimmed milk
4 oz (100 g) chopped banana
2 slices wholemeal toast
low fat spread

7¾ oz (220 g) tin baked beans
2 slices wholemeal toast
1 diet yoghurt

4 oz (100 g) roast chicken
7-9 oz (200-250 g) boiled potatoes
2 oz (50 g) peas or courgettes
2 oz (50 g) carrots or broccoli
1 tablespoon stuffing and gravy
baked apple and sultanas (p. 116)

¼ pt (150 ml) skimmed milk for
    drinks

RECIPES FOR DIET PLANS A B AND C

Leek and carrot soup   (Serves 4)

2½ pt (1.5 litre) chicken stock
1 lb (450 g) trimmed leeks, washed thoroughly and chopped
8 oz (200 g) carrots, peeled and chopped
pinch of ground nutmeg (optional)
salt and pepper to taste

Place the stock, vegetables and nutmeg in a pan, bring to the boil and simmer until the vegetables are tender. Liquidise. Season and serve.

Garden vegetable soup   (Serves 4)

16 fl oz (475 ml) tomato juice
(or a large tin of tomatoes)
1 pt (600 ml) beef or chicken stock
3 oz (75 g) green beans, diced
2 sticks celery, diced
2 medium potatoes, diced
2 medium carrots, diced
½ green pepper, diced
1 medium courgette, diced
salt and pepper to taste

Add the vegetables and seasoning to the tomato juice and stock. Bring to the boil. Simmer until the vegetables are cooked. Serve hot.

Soufflé herb omelette   (Serves 1)

> 2 eggs (separated)
> 1 tablespoon water
> salt and pepper
> 1 teaspoon dried mixed herbs or 1 tablespoon chopped fresh herbs

Beat together the egg yolks, water, salt, pepper and mixed herbs. Whisk egg whites until white and foamy. Fold the egg whites into the egg yolk mixture. Pour the mixture into a non-stick frying pan which has been very lightly greased with oil or butter. Cook over a fast heat until nearly set. Put the pan under the grill for about 2 minutes to brown the top. Serve immediately.

Spanish omelette   (Serves 1)

> 1 oz (25 g) onion, chopped
> 1 oz (25 g) green pepper, chopped
> 2 oz (50 g) mushrooms, chopped
> 4 oz (100 g) tomatoes, chopped
> 2 oz (50 g) cold potato, diced
> 2 oz (50 g) peas
> 2 eggs
> 1 slice wholemeal bread
> low fat spread

In a non-stick frying pan, 'dry' fry the onion and green pepper until soft. Add the mushroom, tomatoes, potatoes and peas and heat through. Beat the eggs and add to the mixture. Cook until set. Serve with the wholemeal bread and low fat spread.

Mushroom omelette   (Serves 1)

> ¼ oz (7 g) margarine
> pulp of 1 tomato
> 2 eggs, beaten
> 2 oz (50 g) mushrooms

Melt the fat in a non-stick frying pan. Beat the tomato pulp into the egg and season. Pour the egg mixture into the pan. When nearly set, add the mushrooms. Serve immediately.

Ratatouille   (Serves 4)

1 tablespoon olive or sunflower oil
2 medium courgettes, sliced ¼ in thick
3 medium tomatoes, quartered, or small tin of tomatoes
1 medium aubergine, cut into 1 in. (2.5 cm) pieces
1 clove garlic, crushed
4 oz (100 g) onions, sliced
1 teaspoon dried mixed herbs or 1 tablespoon chopped fresh herbs

Heat the oil in a large saucepan. Add half the vegetables and sauté for 1-2 minutes. Add the remaining vegetables and sauté for a further minute. Simmer for 15 minutes, stirring occasionally. Add the herbs. Simmer for 20 minutes, stirring occasionally, until the vegetables are soft.

Macaroni cottage cheese   (Serves 2)

½ oz (12 g) sunflower margarine
½ oz (12 g) flour
¼ pt (150 ml) skimmed milk
4 oz (100 g) cottage cheese
handful chives (chopped)
1 teaspoon English mustard or 2 teaspoons French mustard
4 oz (100 g) macaroni
1 oz (25 g) strong Cheddar or Parmesan, grated

Melt the margarine in a pan. Add the flour and stir over a gentle heat for 2 minutes. Take the pan off the heat, gradually add the milk. Replace the pan on the heat and stir until the sauce has thickened. Add the cottage cheese, chives, mustard and half the cheese.

Boil the macaroni for 8-10 minutes. Drain and place in an ovenproof dish. Pour the sauce over the macaroni, top with the remaining cheese and place under the grill until golden.

Fisherman's pie   (Serves 4)

8 oz (200 g) cod or other white fish, cooked and flaked
8 oz (225 g) smoked cod or smoked haddock, flaked
chopped parsley
1 lb (450 g) potatoes, boiled and mashed with a little skimmed milk
2 oz (50 g) Edam cheese, grated

Sauce
1 chopped onion
2 cloves garlic
1 tablespoon oil
15 oz (425 g) can tomatoes
a pinch mixed herbs
salt and black pepper

Sauce
Fry the onion and garlic in oil in a large pan, add tomatoes
and herbs and simmer until sauce thickens, season to taste
with salt and black pepper.

Pie
Pre-heat the oven to gas mark 4, 350°F (180°C).

Put the flaked fish and sauce into an ovenproof dish, mix in
chopped parsley. Spoon or pipe mashed potato over the fish
mixture. Sprinkle top of pie with grated cheese. Bake in the
oven until the top of pie is golden brown.

Pork and pineapple   (Serves 2)

4 oz (100 g) onions, finely chopped
10 oz (250 g) pork tenderloin, cubed
4 oz (100 g) mushrooms, sliced
¼ pt (150 ml) tomato juice
¼ pt (150 ml) chicken stock
4 oz (100 g) pineapple cubes, in natural juice

In a non-stick frying pan, 'dry' fry the onions and pork until
the pork is sealed and the onions are soft. Add the
mushrooms, tomato juice, chicken stock and pineapple cubes.
Simmer for 25-30 minutes. Serve with brown rice.

Sardine and tomato pizza (Serves 4)

Base
2½ fl oz (60 ml) milk
2½ fl oz (60 ml) warm water
1 oz (25 g) sugar
½ oz (15 g) dried yeast
5 oz (125 g) plain wholemeal flour
2 teaspoons oil

Topping
8 oz (200 g) sardines packed in brine
1 small tin chopped tomatoes
2 oz (50 g) mushrooms
½ teaspoon dried or 1 tablespoon fresh oregano

First whisk the sugar and yeast into the milk and warm water. Leave this mixture until it gets a frothy head. Meanwhile sift the flour into a mixing bowl. Pour in the yeast mixture and mix to a dough. Transfer the dough to a working surface and knead for 10 minutes until silky smooth. Replace the dough in a bowl and rub the surface with oil. Cover with cling-film or a damp cloth and put in a warm place to rise for about an hour or until double in size. Knead again for about 5 minutes.

Pre-heat the oven to gas mark 7, 425°F (220°C).

Place the dough in an 8-inch tin and press out to line the tin.

Spread the tomatoes over the base and arrange the mushrooms, tomatoes and oregano on top. Bake for 15-20 minutes.

Tuna pot rice (Serves 1)

4 oz (100 g) cooked brown rice
1 oz (25 g) peas or cucumber
1 oz (25 g) sweetcorn or chopped celery
2 oz (50 g) flaked tuna fish·
1 oz (25 g) green pepper
1 oz (25 g) chopped onion
Squeeze lemon juice
Seasoning
1 tablespoon fresh chopped parsley or other herbs

Mix all ingredients together. Serve cold.

Liver with orange   (Serves 2)

> 1 small onion, chopped
> 2 sticks celery, chopped
> zest and juice of 1 orange
> salt and pepper
> ¼ pt (150 ml) beef or chicken stock
> 8 oz (225 g) ox or lamb's liver, thinly sliced

'Dry' fry the onion and celery until soft. Add the liver and seal. Stir in the zest and juice of the orange, salt and pepper and the stock. Bring to the boil. Simmer gently for about 3 minutes until the liver is cooked.

Grilled chicken rosemary   (Serves 1)

> 8 oz (200 g) chicken joint, skinned
> juice of 1 lemon
> rosemary
> black pepper

Score the top of the chicken joint with a sharp knife and rub with lemon juice, rosemary and black pepper. Brush very lightly with oil and grill for about 15 minutes each side.

Smoked mackerel pâté   (Serves 2)

> 2 oz (50 g) smoked mackerel fillet
> 4 oz (100 g) low fat soft cheese
> 1 tablespoon lemon juice
> 1 tablespoon finely chopped onion
> black pepper to taste

Skin mackerel and flake; add cheese, lemon juice, onion and pepper. Blend all ingredients together until they form a smooth paste. Chill thoroughly and serve with toast or salad.

Chicken and vegetable risotto   (Serves 1)

2 oz (50 g) onion, chopped
2 oz (50 g) green pepper, chopped
2 oz (50 g) peas
4 oz (100 g) brown rice, cooked
½ teaspoon dried oregano or ½ tablespoon chopped fresh oregano
½ teaspoon dried mixed herbs or ½ tablespoon chopped fresh mixed herbs
5 oz (150 g) tinned tomatoes
black pepper
2 oz (50 g) cold cooked chicken, diced
2 oz (50 g) mushrooms, chopped

'Dry' fry the onion until soft. Add the green pepper, peas and rice and fry for a further minute. Add the herbs and tomatoes and season well and simmer for 2 minutes. Add the chicken and mushrooms. Warm through thoroughly and serve.

Chicken curry   (Serves 1)

2 oz (50 g) onion, chopped
4 oz (100 g) cauliflower, chopped
4 oz (100 g) cooking apple, chopped
⅓ pt (200 ml) chicken stock
curry powder, to taste
1 teaspoon lemon juice
1 teaspoon tomato purée
8 oz (200 g) boneless chicken breast, skinned

Simmer the vegetables and apple in the stock with curry powder, lemon juice and tomato purée for 10 minutes. Add the chicken breast. Simmer for 35 minutes until the chicken is cooked. Serve with brown rice.

Beef and vegetable curry   (Serves 4)

8 oz (200 g) onions, chopped
1 lb (400 g) stewing beef, trimmed and cut into cubes
8 oz (200 g) cooking apples, chopped

14 oz (350 g) tinned tomatoes
½ pint (300 ml) beef stock
seasoning
curry powder to taste

'Dry' fry the onions until soft. Add the beef, sprinkle with curry powder and seal. Place all the other ingredients in the pan and simmer together for about 1–1½ hours. Serve with brown rice.

Vegetable and bean hot pot   (Serves 4)

1 large onion, chopped
2 sticks celery, chopped
8 oz (200 g) carrots, peeled and sliced
8 oz (200 g) other vegetables (choose from swede, marrow, cauliflower, parsnip, peppers), peeled and chopped as necessary
15 oz (375 g) tinned tomatoes
15 oz (375 g) tinned red kidney beans, drained
1 lb (450 g) potatoes, scrubbed, boiled and sliced

Put all the vegetables in a pan with a tight-fitting lid. Add the water and bring the contents to a boil. Simmer gently until the vegetables are cooked. Add the tomatoes and beans and bring back to the boil. Turn on the grill. Put the vegetable mixture into a warmed casserole dish and put the sliced potatoes in a layer on top. Grill until brown. Serve immediately.

Note   This dish can be flavoured by the addition of a little chopped bacon or leftover cold meat to the vegetables when the beans and tomatoes are added.

Crunchy fish bake   (Serves 4)

1 lb (450 g) cod/haddock fillets
4 oz (100 g) mushrooms, thinly sliced
4 oz (100 g) onion, sliced
juice of 1 lemon
black pepper
pinch of mixed herbs
2 slices wholemeal bread, toasted and crumbed

Pre-heat the oven to gas mark 4, 350°F (180°C).

Divide the fish into portions and place in the bottom of a shallow casserole. Cover with the mushrooms and onions and pour in the lemon juice. Add the seasonings and cover with foil. Bake for 30 minutes.

Remove the foil. Sprinkle the toasted crumbs over the top. Return to the oven for a further 10 minutes. Serve.

Tuna pasta ribbons (Serves 4)

16 oz (450 g) tinned tomatoes
4 oz (100 g) mushrooms, sliced
4 oz (100 g) green peppers, chopped
4 oz (100 g) onion, chopped
½ oz (15 g) tomato purée
1 clove garlic, peeled and crushed
7 oz (200 g) can tuna fish packed in brine
dried or chopped fresh oregano to taste
black pepper
8 oz (200 g) tagliatelle (pasta ribbons) cooked as directed on the packet

In a pan simmer together the tinned tomatoes, mushrooms, peppers, onion, tomato purée and garlic until the vegetables are soft. Add the tuna and the oregano and black pepper to taste. Add the cooked and well-drained tagliatelle and mix well. Serve.

Beef and beans (Serves 4)

1 lb (450 g) lean stewing beef, cubed
8 oz (200 g) onions, sliced
8 oz (200 g) carrots, diced
18 fl oz (500 ml) beef stock
dried or chopped fresh mixed herbs to taste
black pepper
14 oz (350 g) can baked beans

Pre-heat oven to gas mark 4, 350°F (180°C).

Place beef cubes and vegetables into a casserole dish. Add the stock, herbs and seasoning. Bake for 1 hour. Add the baked beans. Cook for further 30 minutes and serve.

Chunky vegetables and beef   (Serves 4)

8 oz (200 g) onion, chopped
12 oz (300 g) lean mince
8 oz (200 g) fresh or tinned tomatoes, chopped
½ pt (300 ml) beef stock
8 oz (200 g) shredded cabbage
8 oz (200 g) carrot, diced
4 oz (100 g) green pepper, chopped
seasoning

Pre-heat the oven to gas mark 4, 350°F (180°C).
　'Dry' fry the onions until soft. Add the mince and seal. Pour off any fat. Add all the other ingredients. Transfer to a casserole dish. Bake for 30 minutes.

Chilli mince   (Serves 4)

1 lb (400 g) carrots, coarsely grated
1 lb (400 g) lean minced beef
2 medium onions, finely chopped
15 oz (375 g) tin red kidney beans
½ pt (300 ml) beef stock
chilli powder to taste

'Dry' fry the onions until soft. Put in the minced beef and break it up well. Stir until the beef begins to brown. Add the chilli powder, lower the heat and continue cooking, stirring frequently for 2 minutes. Pour off any fat. Mix in the red kidney beans and carrots. Pour in the stock and bring to the boil. Add seasoning and stir well. Cover the saucepan and keep on a low heat for 30 minutes.

Shepherd's pie   (Serves 4)

1 lb (400 g) lean mince
1 onion, chopped
½ pint (300 ml) beef stock
1 oz (50 g) cornflour to thicken

Topping
1 lb (400 g) boiled potatoes, mashed
2 fl oz (40 ml) skimmed milk
¾ oz (20 g) low fat spread

Pre-heat the oven to gas mark 6, 400°F (200°C).

'Dry' fry the onions until soft. Add the meat and seal. Pour off any fat. Add the stock, and cook over a low heat for 30 minutes, stirring from time to time. Mix the cornflour with a tablespoon cold water and then stir into the mince. Simmer until thickened and pour into an ovenproof dish. Mix the skimmed milk and low fat spread into the potatoes. Spoon onto the meat and 'fork' up the top. Bake for about 20 minutes or until golden brown.

Beef casserole   (Serves 4)

2 leeks, sliced
12 oz (300 g) swede
4 oz (100 g) pearl barley
1½ pt (900 ml) beef stock
4 carrots, sliced
1 lb (500 g) lean braising steak, trimmed and cut into strips
a little salt

Put all the ingredients into a saucepan and bring to the boil. Skim the fat from the top of the pan. Stir well and put into a casserole. Cover and cook in a preheated oven (gas mark 3, 325°F, 170°C) for 1½-2 hours or until the meat is tender. Serve hot.

Baked banana and orange   (Serves 1)

1 banana
3½ fl oz (100 ml) orange juice

Pre-heat the oven to gas mark 2, 300°F (150°C).

Peel the banana and place in an ovenproof dish with the orange juice. Bake for 15-20 minutes.

Spicy pear and orange   (Serves 4)

juice of 5 oz (150 g) orange
juice of 1 lemon
¼ teaspoon ground ginger
¼ teaspoon cinnamon
2 tablespoons water
1 lb (450 g) dessert pears, peeled, cored and sliced

In a pan mix the juices with the water and spices, add the pears and bring to the boil and simmer gently until pears are soft. Chill before serving.

Chopped apple crunch   (Serves 1)

5 oz (150 g) dessert apple, chopped
1 slice wholemeal bread, toasted and crumbed, or 2 tablespoons rolled oats toasted in the oven or under the grill

Sprinkle the crumbs or oats over the apple. Serve alone or with natural yoghurt.

Baked apple and sultanas   (Serves 1)

1 medium-sized cooking apple
½ oz (15 g) sultanas
pinch cinnamon

Pre-heat the oven to gas mark 6, 400°F (200°C).
   Wipe the apple and make a shallow cut through the skin around the middle of the apple. Core the apple and fill with sultanas. Sprinkle with cinnamon. Stand in an ovenproof dish. Pour a little water around the apple and bake in the centre of the oven for ¾-1 hour.

DIET PLAN D:
THE EASY WAY

Breakfast every week day

For one person:
Unsweetened muesli with skimmed milk and with a choice of chopped fresh fruit: apple, pear, tangerine, some grapes, a banana or some dried fruit, soaked then cooked and cooled, e.g. apricots or prunes. Coffee or tea, with skimmed milk if you wish but no sugar.

Breakfasts at weekends

For one person:
Orange juice
Choice of small grilled or microwaved kipper.
Smoked haddock fillet, poached in skimmed milk.
Tinned tomatoes on wholemeal toast or sliced fresh tomatoes grilled on wholemeal toast.
Coffee or tea with no sugar.

Day 1

3 oz (75 g) roast chicken breast, sliced with skin removed
5 oz (150 g) new potatoes
3 oz (75 g) broad beans
3 oz (75 g) carrots
gravy – as fat free as possible
apricot fool (p. 127)

2 slices wholemeal bread
low fat spread
2 oz (50 g) cold sliced roast chicken
watercress
1 teaspoon low fat yoghurt as dressing
1 piece fresh fruit

¼ pt (150 ml) skimmed milk for drinks

Day 2

2 slices wholemeal bread
low fat spread
2 oz (50 g) chicken
tomato and cucumber
1 piece fresh fruit

chick pea paprika (p. 122)
2-3 oz (50-75 g) brown rice
1 diet yoghurt

¼ pt (150 ml) skimmed milk for drinks

Day 3

2 slices wholemeal bread
low fat spread
½ can sardines in brine
sliced pickled dill cucumber
1 piece fresh fruit

haddock provençale (p. 124)
5-7 oz (150-200 g) baked potato
mixed salad: lettuce, endive,
    radicchio, Chinese leaves, etc.,
    with low fat yoghurt and herb
    vinegar dressing
fresh fruit salad in natural fruit
    juice

¼ pt (150 ml) skimmed milk for
    drinks

Day 4

2 slices wholemeal bread
low fat spread
2 oz (50 g) lean boiled ham (visible
    fat removed)
French mustard
1 piece fresh fruit

tagliatelle *al limone* (p. 123)
tomato and spring onion salad
    made with 3 small tomatoes with
    low fat yoghurt and herb vinegar
    dressing
5 oz (150 g) natural low fat
    yoghurt mixed with 1 small
    mashed banana
2 teaspoons sultanas

¼ pt (150 ml) skimmed milk for
    drinks

Day 5

2 slices wholemeal bread
low fat spread
1½ oz (40 g) low fat Cheddar-type
    cheese
1 teaspoon tomato pickle
1 piece fresh fruit

tuna and bulgar risotto (p. 126)
salad made with 1 head chicory
    and 1 orange, dressed with low
    fat yoghurt and orange juice
1 piece fresh fruit

¼ pt (150 ml) skimmed milk for
    drinks

Day 6

2 slices wholemeal bread
low fat spread
⅓ medium tin tuna (in brine)
1 tomato, sliced
1 piece fresh fruit

stir-fry beef and noodles (p. 125)
5 oz (150 g) natural low fat
    yoghurt mixed with 1 fresh
    segmented tangerine or satsuma

¼ pt (150 ml) skimmed milk for
    drinks

Day 7

2-egg fresh herb omelette (parsley, chives and tarragon)
1 slice wholemeal bread
1 piece fresh fruit

stuffed sardines (p. 123)
5-7 oz (150-200 g) baked potato
low fat spread
3 oz (75 g) peas
pineapple fool (p. 127)

¼ pt (150 ml) skimmed milk for drinks

Day 8

veal *al limone* (p. 124)
5 oz (150 g) new potatoes
mixed salad: lettuce, radicchio, grated carrot
strips of red pepper with low fat yoghurt and herb vinegar dressing
4-6 oz (100-175 g) fresh fruit salad in natural juice with 1 tablespoon low-fat *fromage frais*

pasta shapes in tomato sauce (p. 121)
1 piece fresh fruit

¼ pt (150 ml) skimmed milk for drinks

Day 9

2 slices wholemeal bread
low fat spread
½ can mackerel in brine with 2 teaspoons low fat yoghurt and 1 teaspoon of capers
1 piece fresh fruit

Chinese fish and noodles (p. 125)
1 piece fresh fruit

¼ pt (150 ml) skimmed milk for drinks

Day 10

2 slices wholemeal bread
low fat spread
1 oz (25 g) pastrami
sliced dill cucumber
1 low fat fruit yoghurt

chicken provençale (p. 124)
5-7 oz (150-200 g) baked potato
3 oz (75 g) sweetcorn
1 piece fresh fruit

¼ pt (150 ml) skimmed milk for drinks

Day 11

2 slices wholemeal bread
low fat spread
1½ oz (40 g) smoked pork loin
1 teaspoon apricot chutney
1 piece fresh fruit

tuna cassoulet (p. 127)
salad of lettuce, Chinese leaves and
   watercress
low fat yoghurt and herb vinegar
   dressing
baked apple, cored and filled with
   raisins

¼ pt (150 ml) skimmed milk for
   drinks

Day 12

2 slices wholemeal bread
low fat spread
2 slices grilled back bacon with fat
   cut off
lettuce and tomato – as much as
   you can fit on
1 teaspoon low fat natural yoghurt
   as dressing
1 low fat fruit yoghurt

chicken and bulgar risotto made
   with brown rice (p. 126)
tomato and spring onion salad
   made with 3 small tomatoes with
   yoghurt and herb vinegar
   dressing
1 piece fresh fruit

¼ pt (150 ml) skimmed milk for
   drinks

Day 13

2 slices wholemeal toast topped
   with 8 oz (225 g) reduced-sugar
   baked beans
1 piece fresh fruit

grilled trout
1 teaspoon Dijon mustard mixed
   with 1 tablespoon low fat
   yoghurt as a sauce
5 oz (150 g) new potatoes
3 oz (75 g) frozen spinach, cooked
   and 1 tablespoon *fromage frais*,
   stirred in off the heat
passion fruit fool (p. 127)

¼ pt (150 ml) skimmed milk for
   drinks

Day 14

5-7 oz (150-200 g) baked potato
¼ oz (10 g) low fat spread
¼ oz (10 g) grated low fat Cheddar
   cheese
1 tablespoon chopped spring
   onions
1 piece fresh fruit

pasta with mushrooms (p. 122)
mixed salad of lettuce, tomatoes,
   cucumber and grated carrot with
   low fat yoghurt and herb vinegar
4-6 oz (100-175 g) fresh fruit salad
   with natural fruit juice

¼ pt (150 ml) skimmed milk for
   drinks

RECIPES FOR DIET PLAN D

Pasta shapes in tomato sauce   (Serves 2)

1 onion, finely chopped
1-2 cloves garlic, finely chopped
1 teaspoon olive oil
14 oz (400 g) tin chopped tomatoes
½ teaspoon dried oregano (or 1 tablespoon finely chopped fresh oregano
or 1 tablespoon finely chopped fresh basil)
4-6 oz (100-175 g) dried pasta shapes such as shells, bows or quills
½ oz (15 g) freshly grated Parmesan cheese

Sauce
Gently fry the onion and garlic in the oil in a non-stick
saucepan. When soft and golden add the tomatoes. Add dried
herbs – if using. Simmer for 10 minutes. Add fresh herbs – if
using.

Pasta
Cook pasta for 12-15 minutes as directed on the packet.
Drain well and add sauce. Stir and serve on heated plates and
sprinkle with Parmesan.

Notes   This amount of sauce makes 2 generous portions with 6 oz
(175 g) pasta as a main course.

The same amount with 6 oz (175 g) pasta will serve 3 people who
want to lose weight more quickly!

Freeze individual portions of this sauce to rustle up quick meals when
you're busy.

Chick pea paprika   (Serves 2)

4 oz (100 g) brown rice
1 onion, finely chopped
1 clove garlic, finely chopped
1 teaspoon olive oil
1 small red pepper, cut into strips
2 teaspoons paprika
14 oz (400 g) can chick peas
14 oz (400 g) can chopped tomatoes
2 tablespoons natural low fat yoghurt

Cook the brown rice in water; it will take approximately 40
minutes. Fry the onion and garlic in the olive oil in a heavy
non-stick saucepan until soft and golden. Add the red pepper
strips and cook a further few minutes. Add the paprika and
stir well. Add the drained chick peas and the chopped
tomatoes. Simmer for 15-20 minutes or until the rice is ready.
Put the yoghurt on top of the chick pea paprika just before
serving (having removed the saucepan from the heat). Drain
the rice and serve as an accompaniment to the chick peas.

Pasta with mushrooms   (Serves 1)

2-3 oz (50-75 g) pasta such as tagliatelle or pasta shapes like shells or
quills
1 clove garlic finely chopped (optional)
3 oz (75 g) mushrooms
1 teaspoon olive oil
1 tablespoon Greek-style yoghurt or low fat *fromage frais*
2 teaspoons finely chopped fresh parsley
¼ oz (10 g) freshly grated Parmesan cheese

Cook pasta as directed on the packet and drain. Cook garlic
and very finely chopped mushrooms in the oil in a non-stick
pan until the mushrooms are very soft. Add the pasta to the
mushrooms with the yoghurt or *fromage frais* and mix well.
Stir in parsley. Serve on heated plate and sprinkle with the
Parmesan.

Tagliatelle al limone (noodles with lemon sauce)   (Serves 1)

2-3 oz (50-75 g) dried tagliatelle or spaghetti (fresh is better and quicker
to cook but more expensive)
½ lemon, zest and juice
½-1 clove garlic, finely chopped (optional)
2 tablespoons of Greek-style yoghurt (sheep or cow's)
¼ oz (10 g) freshly grated Parmesan cheese
black pepper

Cook the pasta as directed on the packet. Peel the zest of the
lemon finely, leaving behind the white pith. Chop finely.
Squeeze the lemon. Add the lemon juice, zest and garlic to the
yoghurt and heat gently. (Unlike normal low fat yoghurt,
Greek-style yoghurt does not separate when heated gently but
do not boil.)

When the pasta is cooked, drain well and add to the lemon
sauce. Mix well. Serve on a heated plate and sprinkle with the
Parmesan and pepper.

Stuffed sardines   (Serves 2)

4 large or 6 medium-sized fresh sardines (or frozen sardines, thawed)
1 clove garlic, finely chopped
1½ oz (40 g) wholemeal breadcrumbs
1 tablespoon finely chopped parsley
1 tablespoon finely chopped sorrel (optional)
½ lemon, juice and zest

Pre-heat the oven to gas mark 6, 400°F (200°C).

Cut the head and tail of each fish. Slit down the stomach
and clean. Place skin side up and run your finger down the
backbone, pressing firmly. You should find that the backbone
and adjoining bones can now be removed. If other small
bones remain, remove them. Mix together the garlic,
breadcrumbs, parsley, sorrel and the juice and finely chopped
zest of the lemon. Stuff the sardines with this mixture and
reshape. Place side-by-side on a large piece of foil and fold
over foil to make a parcel, sealing the edges securely. Cook in
the oven for 25 minutes. Serve with the other half of the
lemon.

Veal al limone (Serves 2)

> 2 x 3-4 oz (75-100 g) veal escalopes
> 1 teaspoon olive oil
> juice of half a large lemon
> 4 tablespoons dry vermouth
> sprigs of parsley

Place the veal escalopes between sheets of greaseproof paper and beat with a steak mallet or a rolling pin until the veal is very thin. Put the oil in a heavy non-stick frying pan and wipe all around the pan with a piece of kitchen paper so there is a thin smear of oil only over the whole surface. Put on the heat and when very hot cook the veal briefly – about 1 minute on each side. Remove and keep warm. Add the lemon juice and the vermouth to the pan. Stir with a wooden spoon to incorporate the juices of the veal. Boil rapidly for about 1 minute, pour over the veal and serve, garnished with the parsley.

Haddock provençale (Serves 4)

> 4 x 5 oz (150 g) boneless and skinless haddock fillets (fresh or frozen)
> 1 quantity of tomato sauce as in pasta shapes in tomato sauce (p. 145)
> 1 oz (25 g) freshly grated Parmesan
> 1 oz (25 g) wholemeal breadcrumbs

Pre-heat the oven to gas mark 6, 400°F (200°C).

Place 2 tablespoons of the tomato sauce on the bottom of an ovenproof dish. Arrange the haddock on top and pour over the rest of the tomato sauce. Mix the cheese and breadcrumbs together and sprinkle over the sauce. Bake in the oven for 25-30 minutes, until the top is browned (35-40 minutes if the haddock is frozen).

Notes Wholemeal breadcrumbs can be made instantly in a food processor. If you don't have one, you can grate bread which is a couple of days old or toast the bread, cool, place in polythene bag and bash with a rolling pin. In this case, add the topping half-way through the cooking time.

For Chicken Provençale use 4 boneless and skinless chicken breasts

For another variation, add 1 finely chopped red or green pepper with the onions and garlic when making the tomato sauce.

Chinese fish and noodles   (Serves 1)

6 oz (175 g) boneless and skinless haddock fillet (or any other white fish) fresh or frozen
1 carrot – cut into matchstick julienne
3 spring onions – shredded to same size as carrots
1 clove garlic, finely chopped
1 teaspoon finely chopped fresh root ginger
1 tablespoon soy sauce
1 tablespoon dry sherry or vermouth
3 oz (75 g) Chinese noodles (preferably wholewheat)

Cut a piece of foil or greaseproof paper big enough to make an envelope for the fish (18 in x 12 in). Place the fish on the foil or paper and sprinkle the carrot, onions, garlic and ginger on top. Combine the soy sauce with the sherry or vermouth and pour on. Fold up the parcel and turn over all the edges several times to make a tight seal. Cook in a hot oven (gas mark 6, 400°F, 200°C) for 10-15 minutes (if fish is frozen for 20-25 minutes).

Serve with the noodles, cooked as directed on the packet.

Note Alternatively this recipe could be cooked in a microwave. You would have to consult your microwave manual for accurate timings, but it should take about 5-7 minutes. Remember, do not use foil in the microwave – use greaseproof paper.

Stir-fry beef and noodles   (Serves 1)

4 oz (100 g) steak – lean with visible fat trimmed off
1 red pepper
½ onion
1 teaspoon soy sauce
1 teaspoon dry sherry or dry vermouth
1 teaspoon tomato purée
1 teaspoon wine vinegar
1 teaspoon oil (preferably sesame oil but otherwise sunflower)
1 clove garlic, finely chopped
1 teaspoon finely chopped fresh root ginger
3 oz (75 g) Chinese noodles (preferably wholewheat)

Cut the beef across the grain into very thin strips. Slice the red pepper and onion into bite-size pieces. Mix together the soy sauce, sherry or vermouth, tomato purée and wine vinegar. Heat the oil in a wok or heavy non-stick frying pan. Add the onion, garlic and ginger and stir-fry for a minute; add the red pepper and continue to stir-fry for a further minute. (Don't cook any longer or the beef will toughen.) Add the soy sauce mixture, bring to the boil, stir well then serve immediately. Serve with the prepared noodles which take about 4 minutes to cook (follow the directions on the packet).

Tuna and bulgar risotto   (Serves 2)

1 onion finely chopped
1 clove garlic finely chopped
1 teaspoon olive oil
4 oz (100 g) bulgar or burghul wheat
2 oz (50 g) frozen peas
7 oz (200 g) can of tuna in brine
½ oz (15 g) Edam cheese, grated

Gently fry onion and garlic in oil in a heavy non-stick frying pan. Add the bulgar wheat and fry gently for a further couple of minutes. Add two cups of water and stir well. Simmer gently until most of the water has been absorbed. Add the peas and tuna and stir until all is hot. Season with salt and pepper. Serve on heated plates and sprinkle with grated cheese.

Note   Bulgar wheat is now available in all supermarkets. It's delicious and takes only a few minutes to cook. But the same dish can be made using brown rice; you will need to keep adding a little water until the rice is cooked, which will take about 40 minutes.

4 oz (100 g) of bulgar wheat or 4 oz (100 g) of brown rice makes a reasonable helping for two; if you're really hungry you could use 3 oz (75 g) of either per person without increasing the calories too much – and that's much better than being tempted to snack or have something sugary later.

Another alternative is to use chopped cooked chicken instead of tuna: about 6 oz (175 g). In this case, you could use chicken stock instead of water.

Tuna cassoulet   (Serves 2)

1 oz (25 g) wholemeal breadcrumbs
½ oz (15 g) freshly grated Parmesan cheese
7 oz (200 g) can of tuna in brine
16 oz (450 g) can of white kidney beans (canellini beans)
½ oz (15 g) onion, finely chopped
1 clove garlic, finely chopped (optional)
8 oz (225 g) canned chopped tomatoes with juice

or

3 fresh tomatoes, skinned chopped and 1 tablespoon tomato purée
mixed with 1 tablespoon of water

Pre-heat the oven to gas mark 6, 400°F (200°C).

Mix together the breadcrumbs and cheese. Combine and
mix well all the other ingredients and place in ovenproof
casserole. Top with breadcrumbs and cheese mixture. Bake in
the oven for 40-45 minutes until the top is browned.

Apricot fool   (Serves 4-6)

4 oz (100 g) dried apricots
8 oz (225 g) low fat *fromage frais*
5 oz (150 g) low fat natural yoghurt

Put the apricots in a small saucepan and cover with water.
Bring to the boil slowly and then simmer gently for 10-15
minutes. Leave to cool. The apricots should absorb most of
the juice.

Finely chop the apricots and their liquid in a liquidiser or
food processor. Add the *fromage frais* and mix. Turn into a
bowl and stir in the low fat yoghurt until thoroughly blended.
Serve in small bowls or glasses topped with a teaspoon of
natural yoghurt.

Note   Alternatives are: *Pineapple Fool* made with 6-8 oz (175-225 g)
fresh pineapple instead of the apricots; or *Passion fruit Fool* made with
the juice and pulp of 4 passion fruits and 4 teaspoons of caster sugar
instead of the apricots.

THE GOURMET PLAN

Breakfast each day
Swiss muesli (p. 133)
¼ pt (150 ml) unsweetened orange or grapefruit juice
tea or coffee, no sugar, skimmed milk if wanted

Day 1
crab salad with coconut – double
helping (p. 142)
1 slice wholemeal bread
1 piece fresh fruit

veal steaks with okra and tomatoes
(p. 143)

¼ pt (150 ml) skimmed milk for
drinks

Day 2
open sandwich with prawns and
salad – lettuce, radicchio or
endive and tomatoes using two
slices wholemeal bread
2 teaspoons low-cal mayonnaise
(p. 149)
1 piece fresh fruit

Blue River trout (p. 146)
4-6 oz (100-175 g) baked potato
mixed salad with low fat yoghurt
dressing
mango yoghurt ice cream (p. 153)

¼ pt (150 ml) skimmed milk for
drinks

Day 3
leek and tomato soup (p. 134)
1 slice wholemeal bread or 1
wholemeal roll
1 piece fresh fruit

steamed poussins with mushroom
and asparagus (p. 148)
2-3 oz (50-75 g) uncooked weight
brown rice
1 piece fresh fruit

¼ pt (150 ml) skimmed milk for
drinks

Day 4
soya bean goulash (p. 144)
1 piece fresh fruit

monkfish with vegetables, Japanese
style (p. 140)
passion fruit curd cake (p. 152)

Day 5

chicken and salad sandwich with
low fat yoghurt dressing (2 slices
wholemeal bread)
1 piece fresh fruit

sea bass with fresh tomato sauce
(p. 137)
4 oz (100 g) steamed potatoes
3 oz (75 g) steamed vegetables
1 piece fresh fruit

¼ pt (150 ml) skimmed milk for
drinks

Day 6

warm calf's liver salad with chives
(p. 144)
1 wholemeal roll
1 piece fresh fruit

beef tartar (p. 145)
mixed salad with low fat yoghurt
dressing
1 wholemeal roll

¼ pt (150 ml) skimmed milk for
drinks

Day 7

egg mayonnaise salad
1 wholemeal roll
1 piece fresh fruit

barbecued hake kebabs with pink
grapefruit (p. 138)
4-6 oz (100-175 g) baked potato
salad with low-cal mayonnaise
(p. 149)
1 piece fresh fruit

¼ pt (150 ml) skimmed milk for
drinks

Day 8

mixed fish soup with vegetables
(p. 134)
1 wholemeal roll or 1 slice
wholemeal bread
1 piece fresh fruit

poached chicken with vegetables
(p. 147)
prune and Armagnac parfait
(p. 152)

¼ pt (150 ml) skimmed milk for
drinks

Day 9

vegetable mosaic slice (p. 135) with
salad
1 slice wholemeal bread
1 piece fresh fruit

salmon with tomato sauce (p. 146)
2-3 oz (50-75 g) brown rice
salad

¼ pt (150 ml) skimmed milk for
drinks

Day 10

lentil salad (p. 142)
1 piece fresh fruit

steamed monkfish with vegetables
(p. 139), with low-cal
mayonnaise (p. 149)
salad
strawberry freshener (p. 133)

¼ pt (150 ml) skimmed milk for
drinks

Day 11

quark soufflé (p. 136)
1 piece fresh fruit

bass in a salt crust (p. 136)
4-6 oz (100-175 g) baked potato
salad

¼ pt (150 ml) skimmed milk for
   drinks

Day 12

tuna and lettuce sandwich with low
   fat yoghurt dressing (2 slices
   wholemeal bread)
1 piece fresh fruit

leek and tomato soup (p. 134)
crab salad with coconut (p. 142)
strawberry freshener (p. 133)

¼ pt (150 ml) skimmed milk for
   drinks

Day 13

2-egg fresh herb omelette
1 wholemeal roll
1 piece fresh fruit

soya bean goulash (p. 144)
4-6 oz (100-175 g) fresh fruit salad

¼ pt (150 ml) skimmed milk for
   drinks

Day 14

prawn salad with low-cal
   mayonnaise (p. 149)
1 piece fresh fruit

vegetable mosaic (p. 135)
warm calf's liver salad with chives
   (p. 144)
1 piece fresh fruit

¼ pt (150 ml) skimmed milk for
   drinks

ANTON MOSIMANN'S RECIPES FOR DIET PLAN E

Swiss muesli   (Serves 4)

  - 4 tablespoons rolled oats
  - 4 fl oz (100 ml) skimmed milk
  - 4 oz (100 g) natural yoghurt (low-fat)
  - 1½ tablespoons lemon juice
  - 2 apples (washed and cored) – 1 red and 1 green
  - 14 oz (400 g) berries (raspberries, strawberries, etc.)
  - 4 tablespoons hazelnuts, toasted, skinned and chopped
  - 4 sprigs of fresh mint
  - 4 raspberries for garnishing

Soak the oats overnight in the milk, then mix with the yoghurt and lemon juice. Grate the apples and add to the mixture. Cut up the berries (if necessary), and add to the mixture. Mix in the chopped nuts, and serve garnished with the mint and raspberries.

Strawberry freshener   (Serves 4)

  - ½ pt (300 ml) low-fat strawberry yoghurt
  - ½ pt (300 ml) buttermilk, chilled
  - 4 strawberries to garnish

Whisk yoghurt and buttermilk together.
   Pour into glasses and top with a fresh strawberry.

Leek and tomato soup   (Serves 4)

7 oz (200 g) leeks, finely cut
7 oz (200 g) onions, finely chopped
7 oz (200 g) tomatoes, deseeded
4 fl oz (120 ml) clear brown stock (p. 150)
1 pt (600 ml) meat broth (p. 141)
salt and freshly ground pepper
a little coarsely chopped parsley for garnish

Sweat the leeks and onions carefully in a non-stick pan until golden, stirring constantly. Add the tomatoes and mix well. Transfer to a saucepan.

Add the clear brown stock and simmer for 5 minutes to reduce a little. Add the meat broth and allow to simmer for 8-10 minutes longer.

Season with salt and pepper and garnish with the parsley before serving.

Note   A vegetable stock or water could be used instead of clear brown stock and meat broth.

Mixed fish soup with vegetables   (Serves 4)

4½ oz (120 g) fillet of sea bass, with skin, carefully boned
3 oz (75 g) fillet of Scottish salmon, with skin, carefully boned
3 oz (75 g) fillet of red mullet, with skin, carefully boned
3 oz (75 g) fillet of turbot, skinned and carefully boned
2 oz (50 g) fillet of sole, skinned and carefully boned
14 fl oz (400 ml) fish stock flavoured with a few strands of saffron (p. 151)
12 baby carrots with stalks, scraped
12 cherry tomatoes, blanched and peeled
8 baby parsnips with stalks, scraped
salt, freshly ground pepper

Cut the fish pieces into small cubes. Season with salt and pepper. Gently heat the fish stock. Meanwhile, steam the vegetables until just tender, and season. Keep warm. Steam the fish pieces over the hot stock for 30 seconds. Arrange the fish and vegetables in four warmed soup plates and then ladle in the hot stock. Serve immediately.

Vegetable mosaic   (Serves 10)

7 oz (200 g) broccoli, cut into tiny florets and stalk diced
6 oz (175 g) spinach, thick stalks removed and washed
8 oz (225 g) large carrots, peeled and sliced
6 oz (175 g) baby corn
5 oz (125 g) courgettes, halved lengthwise
1½ pt (900 ml) vegetable stock from blanching the vegetables
2 tablespoons white herb vinegar
9 leaves of gelatine
fresh chives and carrot leaves or dill to garnish

Sauce
½ pt (300 ml) low fat natural yoghurt
1 tablespoon English mustard
2 tablespoons freshly cut dill
salt and freshly ground pepper

Blanch the broccoli in boiling, salted water. Drain and refresh
in iced water, when cool lay on a towel. Blanch the spinach in
the same water, squeeze dry and cool as above. Cook carrots,
baby corn and courgettes, and cool as above.

Strain the stock through a cloth and measure 1¼ pt (750 ml).
Add the herb vinegar.

Dissolve the gelatine in about a quarter of the vegetable
stock over a gentle heat. Stir in the remaining stock and cool
until the consistency of unbeaten egg white.

Arrange alternate layers of the various vegetables in a 2 pt
(1.25 litre) terrine dish, pouring a little liquid jelly between
the vegetables as you go. Press the last layer below the level of
the liquid.

Chill until set and freeze briefly before unmoulding.

Cut the terrine into slices and allow to soften at room
temperature if necessary.

To make the sauce, mix all the ingredients together, then
chill.

Serve the terrine in slices, garnished with chosen herbs.
Hand the sauce separately.

Note   Any vegetables which are colourful and fresh on the market could
be used in this recipe.

Quark soufflé   (Serves 4)

1¼ lb (500 g) quark
3½ fl oz (100 ml) milk
4 eggs, separated
1 pinch of nutmeg
4 oz (100 g) bacon, diced and sautéed in a non-stick pan
2 tablespoons cornflour
1 tablespoon grated Parmesan
salt and freshly ground pepper

Mix quark, milk, egg yolks, nutmeg and bacon well together.
Season.
  Beat egg whites until almost stiff, add cornflour and beat
again, until stiff. Fold into the quark mixture carefully.
  Line a soufflé dish with non-stick paper and fill with the
quark mixture.
  Sprinkle the Parmesan over.
  Bake in the oven at gas mark 3-4, 325-350°F (170-180°C)
for 55 minutes.

Bass in a salt crust   (Serves 4)

1 x 4 lb (1.75 kg) bass
12 sorrel leaves
2 sprigs dill
2 oz (50 g) parsley
1 bay leaf
4 tomatoes, skinned, seeded and diced
1 bunch chervil, picked into leaves
salt and freshly ground pepper

Salt Crust
2 egg whites
3½ fl oz (100 ml) water
5½ lb (2.5 kg) coarse salt

Pre-heat the oven to gas mark 6, 400°F (200°C).
  Gut the bass through the gills. Remove scales, then fins and
gills with scissors. Wash and pat dry. Stuff with sorrel, dill,
parsley and bay leaf.

To make the crust, beat the egg whites and the water together and, with this, dampen the salt until it forms a sticky paste. Put some of this mixture onto a baking tray large enough to hold the fish. Place the fish on the paste and cover it completely, pressing the mixture well in.

Bake the fish in the oven for 25 minutes. The salt should form into a very hard crust. The steam from the fish is absorbed by the salt.

Knock the salt crust off with a strong tap from a meat mallet and brush off any remaining salt.

Serve with the warmed, diced tomatoes mixed with the chervil and season to taste.

Note Expensive Mediterranean fish (and delicate poultry or best beef) are protected from drying out by a thick salt crust. When in the oven this becomes harder and harder, almost impenetrable. The common bass is often used instead of the more expensive sea bass.

Sea bass with fresh tomato sauce (Serves 4)

4 x 6 oz (175 g) fillets sea bass, with skin, scaled and carefully boned
flour to dust fish
1 quantity tomato coulis (p. 141)
1 bunch of spring onions, cut into pieces 1 in (2.5 cm) long
1½ oz (40 g) butter
1 tablespoon olive oil
salt, freshly ground pepper and pinch of sugar

Season the bass fillets with salt and pepper and dust with flour. Set aside.

Make the tomato coulis (p. 141). Keep warm.

Sauté the spring onions in a non-stick pan with a little water until tender. Season with salt, pepper and sugar. Remove, drain and keep warm.

Sauté the bass fillets in the butter and oil for about 3 minutes on each side. Drain on kitchen towel.

To serve, spoon the sauce on to four warmed plates and place the fish fillets on top. Garnish with the spring onions.

Barbecued hake kebabs with pink grapefruit   (Serves 4)

1½ lb (675 g) fillets of hake, skinned, carefully boned, and rolled up neatly
3 pink grapefruit, skinned and segmented
4 teaspoons groundnut oil
1 fennel bulb, the 'layers' separated, cut into ¾ in (1.5 cm) pieces and blanched
1 medium onion, the 'layers' separated, cut into ¾ in (1.5 cm) pieces and blanched
4 medium tomatoes, blanched, skinned, cut into quarters and deseeded

Marinade
1 clove of garlic
8 fl oz (250 ml) tomato juice
a dash of sherry
a dash of soy sauce
the juice of 1 lemon
salt

Sauce
4 oz (100 g) plain yoghurt
a dash of Angostura bitters
1 tablespoon dill, finely cut
1 tablespoon chives, finely cut
salt, freshly ground pepper

Mix together all the marinade ingredients and pour over the prepared fish rolls. Leave for 4 hours, occasionally turning the fish in the marinade. Remove the fish and pat dry with kitchen towel. Cut into 1 in (2.5 cm) pieces.

Thread the fish securely on to skewers, alternating with grapefruit segments, and brush with groundnut oil. Thread the fennel, onion and tomato alternately on skewers and brush with groundnut oil.

Lightly grill all the kebabs over charcoal for about 10 minutes, turning occasionally.

Meanwhile mix all the ingredients together for the sauce. Season to taste.

Serve the fish and grapefruit kebabs with the vegetable kebabs, and the sauce separately.

Braised lentils with vegetables   (Serves 4)

1 large onion
½ oz (10 g) butter
4 oz (100 g) carrots
4 oz (100 g) leeks
2 tomatoes, peeled and diced
½ clove garlic, crushed
1 sprig thyme
18 fl oz (500 ml) chicken stock
8 oz (225 g) brown dried lentils, soaked
8 oz (225 g) potatoes, finely diced
4 tablespoons red wine
1 tablespoon red wine vinegar
salt, freshly ground pepper

Sweat the chopped onion in butter for 2 to 3 minutes. Cut the carrots and leeks into thin strips and sweat with onions. Add the tomatoes, crushed garlic, thyme and sauté for 1 to 2 minutes.

Add 9 fl oz (250 ml) of chicken stock.

Simmer the drained lentils in the remaining stock for 45 minutes. Remove 1 cup of lentils and liquidise.

10 minutes before serving mix in potatoes, red wine, vinegar, lentils and vegetables and continue to simmer.

Season with salt and pepper.

Steamed monkfish with vegetables   (Serves 4)

1 lb 14 oz (800 g) monkfish, boned and skinned
1 clove of garlic, cut into fine slivers
1 bouquet garni
2 medium size onions
2 cloves
9 oz (250 g) carrots, peeled and cut in slices
2 medium size leeks, cut in slices
2 small white radishes, cut in slices
1 small celeriac, peeled
salt, freshly ground pepper

Spike the fish with the garlic.

Put the bouquet garni and the onions stuck with the cloves in salted water and bring to the boil. Add the vegetables, cook *al dente*, and keep warm.

Steam the fish for 7 minutes over the water in which the vegetables were cooked.

Cut the monkfish in slices and serve arranged over the vegetables.

Monkfish with vegetables, Japanese style   (Serves 4)

   1 lb (450 g) fillet of monkfish, skinned
   1 lemon, juiced
   salt and freshly ground pepper
   2 oz (50 g) Daikon (white radish)
   2 oz (50 g) red radish
   2 oz (50 g) carrot
   1 oz (25 g) celery
   2 tablespoons Meaux mustard
   2 tablespoons Dijon mustard
   2 tablespoons rice vinegar
   4 tablespoons fish stock (p. 151)
   1 tablespoon flaked almonds, toasted
   4 small bunches of lamb's lettuce

Slice the monkfish very thinly, and season with lemon juice, salt and pepper. Leave to marinate for 5-10 minutes in a cool place.

Cut radish, carrot and celery into julienne strips.

Meanwhile mix the two mustards, vinegar and fish stock together. Season well and leave to stand at room temperature.

Just before serving, mix the mustard sauce together and spoon over the fish. Garnish with the julienne of vegetables, flaked almonds and lamb's lettuce.

Tomato coulis   (Serves 10)

1 oz (25 g) unsalted butter
1 small onion, chopped
2 lb (1 kg) ripe red tomatoes, deseeded and chopped
1 clove garlic, crushed
bouquet garni
1 teaspoon (5 ml) sugar
2 tablespoons (30 ml) tomato purée (optional)
salt, freshly ground pepper

Melt the butter in a saucepan and cook the onion until soft but not coloured.

Add the tomatoes, garlic, bouquet garni, sugar and salt and pepper to taste and simmer uncovered for 30-40 minutes or until sauce is thick.

Work the sauce through a strainer and return to the pan.

Re-heat and if necessary reduce it. It should be the consistency of thin cream. Purée in a food processor for 5-10 minutes to make it very smooth.

If a deeper colour is desired, add the tomato purée.

Meat broth   Yield: 1¾ pt (1 litre)

2 lb (1 kg) beef bones, chopped
7 oz (200 g) lean beef trimmings
2 oz (50 g) bouquet garni
½ onion, browned
2½ pt (1·5 litre) water
salt and freshly ground pepper

Soak the beef bones in cold water, then blanch.

Place the bones and beef trimmings in cold water and bring to the boil. Skim.

Add the remaining ingredients. Simmer for 2 hours, occasionally skimming and removing the fat.

Strain broth through a cloth or fine sieve and season to taste.

Note In order to give the broth a good colour, the onion is browned in its skin under a grill, on the hotplate or in a roasting tin in the oven.

Lentil salad (Serves 4)

5 oz (150 g) brown lentils
1 small leek, cut into fine strips
1¾ pt (1 litre) vegetable stock (p. 149)
1 small onion, finely chopped
1 teaspoon thyme, finely chopped
4 teaspoons white wine vinegar
1 teaspoon French mustard
8 teaspoons safflower oil
4 oz (100 g) button mushrooms, thinly sliced
juice of ½ lemon
salt, freshly ground pepper

Cook the lentils and leek in the stock.

Meanwhile make a salad dressing by mixing together the onion, thyme, wine vinegar, mustard and safflower oil. Marinate the mushrooms in lemon juice and add to the salad dressing.

When the lentils and leeks are cooked *al dente*, drain them well and add them to the salad while still warm. Season and mix carefully.

Let the salad rest for 2 hours before serving.

Note It is important that the lentils are fresh, i.e. from the last crop. Any pulse which is years old is difficult to cook to be tender.

Crab salad with coconut (Serves 4)

8 oz (225 g) white crab meat
1 small shallot, finely chopped
1 tomato, blanched, skinned, deseeded and cut into thin strips
1 stick of celery, trimmed and cut into thin strips
2 oz (50 g) fine green beans, trimmed, blanched and cut into strips
1 oz (25 g) fresh coconut, shredded
juice of ½ lemon
1 grapefruit, peeled, pith removed and segmented (reserve juice)
1 orange, peeled, pith removed and segmented (reserve juice)
salt, freshly ground pepper
chervil sprigs to garnish

Mix together the crab meat, shallot, tomato and celery strips, green beans and coconut. Moisten with the lemon, orange and grapefruit juices and season to taste with salt and pepper.

Arrange the fruit segments on four plates, spoon the crab mixture on top and garnish with chervil sprigs. Serve well chilled.

Veal steaks with okra and tomatoes   (Serves 4)

8 x 1½ oz (40 g) veal steaks or escalopes
salt and freshly ground pepper
9 oz (250 g) quark
¾ oz (20 g) horseradish, grated
2 tablespoons parsley, chopped
2 fl oz (50 ml) clear brown stock (p. 150)
3 fl oz (85 ml) cider
¼ oz (10 g) shallots, finely chopped
5½ oz (165 g) saffron rice
3½ oz (90 g) okra, cooked
3½ oz (90 g) tomato fillets
1 tablespoon mixed fresh herbs, chopped, for garnish

Beat the steaks thinly and season them.

Season the quark with horseradish and parsley. Spread the quark on the veal slices, roll them and bind them with thread.

Sauté the paupiettes all round in a non-stick pan carefully. Add 2 spoons of the stock and cover pan until done. Remove the paupiettes from pan, keep warm.

Add the cider and remaining meat broth and reduce to required consistency.

Sauté shallots in a non-stick pan.

Place the paupiettes on hot saffron rice

Serve warmed okra and tomatoes as garnish; and sprinkle over the fresh herbs.

Note To make tomato fillets:
Skin and seed a large tomato and cut into quarters. Slice each quarter lengthwise in 4.

Warm calf's liver salad with chives   (Serves 4)

8 oz (225 g) dandelion leaves or 1 curly endive well washed and torn
4 small tomatoes, skinned and seeded
7 oz (200 g) calf's livers, trimmed
2 tablespoons freshly cut chives

Yoghurt dressing
4 oz (100 g) low fat natural yoghurt
2 teaspoons mild wine vinegar
2 teaspoons light soya sauce, or to taste
1 teaspoon fresh yeast
2 teaspoons mixed fresh herbs, cut (such as parsley, dill, basil)
2 teaspoons onion, finely chopped
1 sliver of garlic, crushed
½ teaspoon English mustard
salt and freshly ground pepper

For the dressing, mix all the ingredients together until evenly
blended and season to taste. Pour a little of the dressing on to
four individual plates. Arrange the salad leaves on top.

Cut the tomatoes into julienne strips.

Season the calf's livers and sauté in a non-stick pan until
lightly browned on all sides, but still pink in the centre.

Arrange liver on the salad leaves and sprinkle with tomato
julienne and chives. Serve the salad at once, with the
remaining yoghurt dressing passed separately.

Soya bean goulash   (Serves 4)

8 oz (225 g) soya beans (dried)
2 pt (1.2 litre) water
8 oz (225 g) mushrooms
2 medium onions, thinly sliced
1 large clove garlic, finely chopped
1 tablespoon paprika
2 teaspoons caraway seeds
1½ oz (40 g) tomatoes, skinned, seeded and diced
¾ pt (450 ml) vegetable stock (p. 149)
1 bay leaf
2 tablespoons chopped parsley
2 large pickled gherkins, rinsed and chopped

Soak the soya beans and simmer them for 3 hours, drain them if necessary.

Pre-heat the oven to gas mark 3, 325°F (170°C).

Thinly slice the mushrooms.

In a non-stick pan, gently cook the onions and garlic, adding a few spoons of vegetable stock to prevent sticking. When soft, add paprika and caraway, tomato dice and vegetable stock. Bring to the boil, add beans and mushrooms and bay leaf.

Transfer to an ovenproof casserole, cover and put it into the oven for 20 minutes.

Add the parsley and gherkins for the final 3 minutes of cooking time.

Beef tartar   (Serves 4)

4 oz (100 g) quark
1 tablespoon milk
4 round slices of bread, toasted
14 oz (400 g) lean beef, sirloin, minced
1 egg yolk
1 tablespoon Cognac
1 teaspoon shallots, finely chopped
a few drops Worcestershire sauce
4 onion rings
12 capers, rinsed
salt, freshly ground pepper

Mix quark, milk and season with salt and pepper, spread the mixture on the bread slices.

Mix together the beef, egg yolk, Cognac, shallots and Worcestershire sauce and spread on top of the quark.

Garnish each with 1 onion ring and place 3 capers in the middle of each onion ring.

Serve immediately.

Blue River trout   (Serves 4)

Court Bouillon
7 fl oz (200 ml) water
8 fl oz (250 ml) white wine
5 fl oz (150 ml) vinegar
2 oz (50 g) salt
2 onions, finely chopped
1 leek, finely chopped
1 carrot, finely chopped
1 small bunch parsley
pepper, bay leaf, thyme
juice of 1 lemon

4 very fresh river or rainbow trout
5 oz (125 g) fromage blanc or quark
4 teaspoons fresh mixed herbs (parsley, chervil, chives), chopped slices of
lemon to garnish

Make a strong Court Bouillon from all the ingredients and
allow to boil gently for about 15 minutes. Add the gutted and
cleaned trout to the boiling broth, lower to a gentle heat and
allow to simmer for about 10 minutes (do not boil).

Mix the fromage blanc or quark with the herbs and season
to taste.

Very carefully lift the trout out of the liquid, and arrange on
warm plates. Divide the fromage blanc between the four
plates. Garnish with slices of lemon and serve immediately.

Note   The fish must be very very fresh and should be handled as little as
possible to retain the slime on the skin which goes blue as it is cooked.

Salmon with tomato sauce   (Serves 4)

1½ lb (750 g) salmon, skinned and filleted
salt and freshly ground pepper

Tomato sauce
14 oz (400 g) firm, ripe tomatoes, blanched and skinned
4 teaspoons reduced vegetable stock (p. 149)
1 teaspoon Dijon mustard
1 small clove of garlic, peeled and crushed

1 teaspoon each of chopped parsley and finely cut tarragon, coriander leaves and chervil
8 coriander leaves
salt and freshly ground pepper

As the tomatoes in the sauce are only heated, not cooked, they retain their vitamins fully.

To make the sauce, halve the tomatoes crosswise, remove the seeds and chop the flesh into tiny dice.
  Mix together the reduced stock, mustard, garlic and herbs. Stir in the tomato dice and season to taste with salt and pepper.
  Season the salmon with salt and pepper, then grill for 3-4 minutes.
  Heat the sauce very gently in a bowl over hot water.
  Put the slightly warm sauce on four individual plates. Arrange the fillets of fish on top and serve immediately. Garnish with coriander leaves.

Poached chicken with vegetables (Serves 4)

1 × 4¾ lb (2.2 kg) chicken, preferably maize-fed, cut into 8 pieces
3½ pt (2 litres) chicken stock
1 onion stuck with cloves
1 bayleaf
2 cloves garlic, peeled
6 white peppercorns
1 bunch fresh herbs (rosemary, thyme, parsley stalks)
4 pieces celery, about 2 in. (5 cm) in length
4 pieces leek, about 2 in. (5 cm) in length
4 small carrots, peeled
4 small onions, skinned
5 ozs (120 g) broccoli, cut into florets
8 cabbage leaves

Bring a large saucepan of water to the boil. Add the chicken and bring back to the boil. Drain and allow to cool slightly.
  In a large pan, boil up the stock, onion, bayleaf, garlic peppercorns and herbs. Simmer for 20 minutes. Add the chicken and poach for 10 minutes. Remove the chicken and skin the pieces when cool enough to handle.

Strain the stock and remove all traces of fat with kitchen paper.

Return the chicken and stock to a clean pan and add the celery, leeks, carrots, onions, broccoli and cabbage. Bring to the boil and simmer for 10-15 minutes until cooked.

Strain the chicken and vegetables and keep warm.

Boil the chicken stock rapidly to reduce by half. Adjust seasoning to taste.

Arrange the cabbage leaves in four soup plates and place the chicken and vegetables on top. Pour over some stock and garnish with thyme. Serve at once.

Steamed poussins with mushroom and asparagus   (Serves 4)

5½ oz (165 g) chicken meat, boned
7 oz (200 g) sweetbreads
2 oz (50 g) onions, finely chopped
4½ oz (120 g) mushrooms, diced
2 oz (50 g) oyster mushrooms, stalks removed
salt, freshly ground pepper
18 fl oz (500 ml) white poultry stock (p. 150)
4 baby chickens (poussins)
1 oz (25 g) carrots, cut into strips
1½ oz (40 g) asparagus tips, blanched
1½ oz (40 g) haricot beans, blanched
8 button onions, blanched
4 oyster mushrooms for garnish, stalks removed

Remove the skin from the chicken meat and sweetbreads and trim.

Sauté the chopped onions in a non-stick pan, add the mushrooms, sweetbreads and chicken meat and season. Add the chicken stock and simmer slowly. Remove the sweetbreads, chicken meat and mushrooms from the stock, allow to cool and cut into small cubes.

Greatly reduce the stock, to moisten the finely chopped sweetbreads, chicken meat and mushrooms. Mix all together well, season and stuff the chickens with the mixture.

Wrap the chickens in aluminium foil and cook over steam for about 30 minutes. In the last 5 minutes add the remaining vegetables to the steamer to reheat.

Remove the skin from the chickens, and serve.

Low-cal mayonnaise   (Serves 4)

1 raw egg
½ clove of garlic
2 small shallots
1 teaspoon lemon juice
1 teaspoon French mustard
1 shelled, hard-boiled egg
4 oz (100 g) low fat yoghurt
salt and freshly ground pepper
fresh herbs – chives, basil, chervil, dill or parsley – finely chopped

Mix all ingredients except hard-boiled egg, yoghurt and herbs, in a blender. Add the hard-boiled egg and blend until smooth.

Remove from blender container and fold in the yoghurt. Stir in the herbs. Season well and keep cool.

Vegetable stock   Yield: 1¾ pt (1 litre)

1¼ oz (30 g) unsalted butter
1½ oz (40 g) onions
1½ oz (40 g) leeks
¾ oz (20 g) celery
1¼ oz (30 g) cabbage
¾ oz (20 g) fennel
1¼ oz (30 g) tomatoes
2½ pt (1.5 litre) water
½ bay leaf
½ clove
salt and freshly ground pepper

Cut up and finely chop vegetables.

Melt the butter and sweat the onions and leeks in it. Add the remaining vegetables and sweat for a further 10 minutes.

Add the water, bay leaf and clove. Simmer for 20 minutes.

Strain through a cloth or fine sieve, remove all traces of fat with kitchen paper and season to taste.

Note   This is usually used for soups and vegetarian dishes.

White poultry stock   Yield: 1¾ pt (1 litre)

1 boiling fowl or chicken bones (blanched)
3½ pt (2 litre) water
2 oz (50 g) white bouquet garni (onions, white of leek, celeriac and herbs)
salt and freshly ground pepper

Put the boiling fowl or bones in a saucepan, fill up with cold water, bring to the boil and skim. Add the bouquet garni and seasoning.

Leave to simmer carefully for 2 hours, occasionally skimming and removing the fat.

Strain the stock through a fine cloth or sieve and season to taste.

Note   The boiling fowl can afterwards be used for various cold dishes.

Clear brown stock   Yield: 1¾ pt (1 litre)

2 lb (1 kg) veal bones and trimmings, cut in small pieces
¾ fl oz (20 ml) groundnut oil
2 oz (50 g) mirepoix (diced carrots, onions, turnips and celery)
1¼ lb (500 g) tomatoes, diced
4½ pt (2.5 litres) water
salt and freshly ground pepper

Pre-heat the oven to gas mark 8, 450°F (230°C).

Roast the veal bones and trimmings with the oil in a roasting pan in the oven until brown.

Remove the oil with a spoon or strain off, add the mirepoix and tomatoes and roast for another 4 to 5 minutes. Remove from the oven and transfer to a saucepan.

Add ½ pt (300 ml) water and bring to the boil. Reduce to a glaze.

Repeat 4 times.

Add the remaining water and simmer for 2 hours, occasionally skimming and removing the fat.

Strain through a cloth or fine sieve and season to taste.

Fish stock Yield: 1¾ pt (1 litre)

2 lb (1 kg) broken up fish bones and trimmings
2 oz (50 g) white mirepoix (onions, white of leek, celeriac, fennel leaves, dill)
1¼ oz (30 g) mushroom trimmings
¾ oz (20 g) unsalted butter
7 fl oz (200 ml) white wine
2 pt (1.2 litre) water
salt and freshly ground pepper

Thoroughly wash the fish bones and trimmings.

Sweat the mirepoix and the mushroom trimmings in the butter. Add the fish bones and trimmings, white wine and water.

Simmer for 20 minutes, occasionally skimming and removing the fat. Strain through a cloth or fine sieve and season with salt and pepper.

Note In order to produce a good fish stock, only the bones of fresh white fish (sole, turbot) should be used.

Passion fruit sauce (Serves 4)

6 passion fruit
2 oz (50 g) sugar or to taste
½ pt (300 ml) water
¼ orange, juiced
¼ oz (10 g) arrowroot
1 fl oz (25 ml) water

Cut the fruit in half and scoop out the seeds and pulp into a small bowl.

Put the fruit shells, sugar and water into a pan and simmer for 20 minutes. Strain and discard the shells.

Add the seeds and pulp of the fruit to the syrup and simmer for 3 minutes. Add the orange juice to taste.

Mix the arrowroot and 1 fl oz (25 ml) water together and use enough to thicken the sauce by bringing it just to the boil.

Strain the sauce through a fine sieve.

Serve lukewarm.

Prune and Armagnac parfait   (Serves 4)

½ pt (300 ml) weak strained tea
8 oz (225 g) prunes
½ pt (300 ml) thick, low fat yoghurt
3 tablespoons (45 ml) Armagnac
2 egg whites
¼ pt (150 ml) low fat fromage frais

Simmer the prunes in a little tea until soft. When cool enough to handle, remove the stones. Place the prunes in a liquidiser with the yoghurt and Armagnac and blend to a purée.

Whisk the egg whites until stiff.

Mix the fromage frais into the prune mixture, then fold in the whisked egg whites. Pour into a container and freeze. Just before it is completely frozen, whisk the parfait thoroughly and return it to the freezer in a container deep enough to scoop from.

Remove the parfait from the freezer 20 minutes before serving to allow it to soften sufficiently.

Passion fruit curd cake   (Serves 8)

2 tablespoons clear honey
4 eggs, separated
1 lb (450 g) ricotta cheese, or sieved cottage cheese
6 passion fruit
4 oz (100 g) ground almonds
2 oz (50 g) fine semolina
oil to grease tin

Pre-heat oven to gas mark 5, 375°F (190°C).

Lightly grease a shallow 8 in (20 cm) springform cake tin.

Place the honey and egg yolks in a bowl and whisk until thick and creamy. Whisk in the cheese and pulp of the fruit. Add the almonds and the semolina, and mix together well.

Whisk the egg whites until stiff and fold in.

Pour into the prepared tin and bake for 25 minutes, until firm and set. Remove from the oven and allow to cool before removing from the tin.

Serve with Passion Fruit Sauce (p. 151) if desired.

Mango yoghurt ice cream   (Serves 4)

8 oz (200 g) mangoes, peeled and stoned
¾ oz (20 g) caster sugar
11 oz (300 g) low-fat yoghurt
2 egg yolks
1 oz (25 g) caster sugar
3 tablespoons water

Purée mangoes in a food processor and mix with the caster sugar and yoghurt.

Beat the egg yolks until creamy.

Boil the 1 oz (25 g) of sugar and water together until the bubbles settle and flatten.

Using an electric whisk turned on full, gradually pour the hot syrup into the egg yolks, in a small bowl, and keep beating until the mixture is cold and thick.

Stir the egg-yolk cream with the yoghurt mixture, put into a 18 fl oz (500 ml) mould and freeze for 2-3 hours, whisking the ice vigorously from time to time. Before serving, allow to thaw in the refrigerator for 20 minutes.

Note   Strawberries or raspberries could be used as an alternative to mangoes.

EATING OUT

There are two ways of approaching a meal out when you're on the BBC Diet: controlling yourself or letting yourself go.

If you've gone out for a special occasion, I see no problem in having anything you want to eat. Why not enjoy yourself to the full? You can be 'off' your diet for one night and then back on it again the next day.

On the other hand, if you have to eat out often, you can't afford to take this liberal attitude – meals out two or three times a week can wreak havoc with your diet. Or you may feel that the fleeting enjoyment of a meal isn't worth delaying the day you reach your ideal weight.

If you're going out to a friend's house, it's sensible to say when you're accepting the invitation that you don't want to eat too much fattening food. This may be a challenge to a friend who's a keen cook to come up with something pleasing and low in calories – maybe you could send an advance present of a copy of *The BBC Diet*! If you are faced with food you'd rather not eat too much of, do remember how discouraging it is if you've been slaving over cooking to have someone refuse food. Your tactic in this situation should not be to refuse, but ask for a small helping. If you really get a small helping, you can eat it all; if you don't you can leave some. Obviously, don't add things like butter to your bread or cream to your pudding. Above all, remember that you can make up for a few hundred calories too many over the following week. I can't emphasise enough that it's what we eat *most* of the time that makes us fat, not what we eat occasionally.

If you're going to eat in a restaurant then obviously you're more in control. Before you go, it's a good idea to read through the guidelines so they're fixed in your mind. Here are some other thoughts that can flash through it as you read the menu:

- Steer clear of alcohol: apart from the calories it encourages you to eat more. Remember how chic a mineral water is with ice and lemon.
- Don't eat the nibbles with the drinks.
- You should be able to spot a low-calorie first course – melon, grapefruit, clear soup are all perfect choices. As you look at each item ask yourself, 'Does this contain fat?' (perhaps even 'Does this contain sugar?'!) Remember avocado is quite high

in calories and usually comes with an oily dressing. Humus and taramasalata are usually full of oil. If there is something 'salady' make sure you ask if you can have it without the dressing.

- Ask for wholemeal bread; don't be tempted to put butter on it.
- For your main course you should, on the whole, look for something as simple as possible. The general rule is – the more human ingenuity has been at work on it, the more calories it contains (unless your chef follows Anton Mosimann's principles of *cuisine naturelle, naturellement*).

  Choose grilled fish, grilled chicken or a small grilled steak. Cut off the chicken skin and any visible fat on the steak. Make sure that you say you want it absolutely plain (ask for a slice of lemon to flavour it); make sure *maître d'* or any other kind of butter goes nowhere near it.
- Ask for a baked potato, or new potatoes, without added butter. You could try asking for low-fat yoghurt or low-fat spread for your baked potato. Boiled rice is a possibility. Make sure also your vegetables come neat – ask beforehand as often they come swimming in fat. If you're having a salad, again stress that you don't want any dressing. Trust your lemon slice again.
- For dessert, your best bet is fresh fruit. All restaurants should be able to provide this. Fresh fruit salad (no cream) would be an alternative but it's often quite sugary. Sorbet would be another reasonable bet. Avoid cheese – you'd probably eat too much. Of course, you're not even going to look at a sweet trolley.
- Don't put cream in your coffee. Often this is all that is offered. Ask for skimmed milk – you should get ordinary milk at least.
- Don't start nibbling the mints or chocolates they bring with the coffee.
- If you're having an Indian or Chinese meal, you should do well as the eating is usually communal. Make sure you have plain boiled rice and just taste small helpings of the other dishes.

ENTERTAINING

Entertaining at home is easier than eating out because you're in complete control. It is possible to give your guests healthy, slimming food without their knowing it – just look at some of Anton Mosimann's recipes. If you entertain the same people regularly, you should certainly be concerned that what you're giving them is reasonably healthy. It's also helping you to stick to your diet while tucking in with abandon. Either follow recipes which you know are low in calories (like Anton's) or adapt them so that they conform to the BBC Diet guidelines (see below).

If, on the other hand, you want to give your guests a real blow-out, make sure you leave somewhere in the meal to retreat to!

- serve carrot, pepper and celery sticks as alternative nibbles with drinks
- serve sauces and dressings separately so you don't need to have them. The same goes for butter and cream.
- always serve fresh fruit as well as calorific puddings so you (or others) can say, 'I'm full but can manage a few grapes.' Fresh fruit salad in unsweetened fruit juice is the alternative.

Adapting recipes

If you keep 'thinking fat and thinking sugar' you should be able to adapt many of your favourite recipes so that they contain far fewer calories.

- Gradually cut down the amount of sugar you add in recipes and aim to get down to half your normal quantity of sugar.
- Cutting the fat and the sugar in half works in most baking recipes.
- Substitute skimmed milk for whole milk and fromage frais or low-fat natural yoghurt for cream. (If you're heating yoghurt, remember that a teaspoon of cornflower mixed with milk and stirred in should ensure that it doesn't curdle.)
- In all chicken recipes remove the skin.
- Always choose lean meat and trim off the fat.
- With soups, stocks and casseroles always try to prepare in advance. If you leave them to cool, the fat rises to the top and can then be spooned off.
- After frying, pour off any fat and perhaps blot it up also with kitchen paper.
- But, preferably, of course you won't be frying! Think – can I grill? If not, dry-fry in a heavy non-stick frying pan. If that's not possible, stir-fry in minimal oil and blot up the excess later.

- Whenever there's fat in a recipe ('1 oz (25 g) of butter', '4 tbsp of oil'), always halve it, at least. Better still, try it without.

MAINTAINING YOUR IDEAL WEIGHT

At last, you've reached your goal – the new, slim you. Think of your achievement as an investment – you don't want to throw it away by starting to get fat again.

- If you've followed the BBC Diet, you'll now have a great practical knowledge of why we put on weight and how we can lose it. Applying that knowledge is your insurance policy against getting fat again.
- Monitor your weight carefully. Weigh yourself once a week. Remember that fat creeps up slowly, pound by pernicious pound. If we only put on 4 oz (100 g) a week – that's nearly a stone (7.25 kg) in a year.
- By following the BBC Diet, you will have become used to low-fat, low-sugar, high fibre food; you'll have discovered that it's enjoyable. Hopefully, some of the new food habits you've developed will have become ingrained and will last a lifetime. Remember that although the BBC Diet is the very best diet for losing weight, it's also the very best for becoming healthy and keeping healthy. Try to incorporate as many of its guidelines into your life 'post-diet' – and remember, getting your family and particularly your children into healthy eating ways is one of the biggest gifts you can give them.
- If you read through the guidelines 'Where's the Fat?', 'Where's the Sugar?' and 'Where's the Fibre?' (see pages 67-71) again, you'll see that some of them suggest modifications you can make once you've gained your ideal weight. If you find yourself putting on weight again, you need to go back to the original guidelines for a while; following them strictly for a few days will lose the extra couple of pounds.
- What if you can't face life without chocolate, cream cakes, fish and chips? Don't despair. Remember that *no* food can make you fat if you only eat it once a week. What you eat most of the time is what makes you fat, not what you eat occasionally. Eat sensibly, trying to follow the guidelines for six (or better six and a half) days a week and then eat what you fancy for one or two meals a week. Of course, you could find that healthy food becomes your favourite food – it does happen!

- Whatever you do, don't creep back into bad habits that you don't even get much pleasure from – an extra tablespoon of oil here, a teaspoonful of sugar there. Eat slim 90 per cent of the time – feast for 10 per cent. That should be your motto for life.
- Enjoy the 'rewards' you've earned; you may build in others every few months to help maintain the new slim you.

CHAPTER 8

THE BBC DIET – THE THIRD STEP: EXERCISE

Exercise is an integral part of the BBC Diet. It will help you in so many ways to lose those excess pounds and to get to your ideal weight quicker and in better shape. If you did nothing at all to your diet and just started regular exercise which gradually became more vigorous, you would lose weight. It might take you a long time, though, to get down to your target weight. The combination of the BBC Diet and exercise is the very best – and healthiest – way to lose weight. For just as you should consider some of the dietary changes you've made on the BBC Diet as changes for life, so from now you should be determined that exercise – enjoyable exercise! – should be a regular part of your life. It will be one of the main planks in helping you to *stay* slim and also, as we'll see, will give you so many other benefits.

EXERCISE IS NORMAL

We saw in Chapter Three that one of the reasons that being overweight is now more common than in our grandparents' day is that we are all so much less physically active.

The human body is designed to need regular exercise. Our cave-people ancestors had regular exercise: they ran and climbed in order to hunt and gather food. Everyone, in every generation but our own, took physical activity for granted. Now we live in a push-button world, in which we don't even have to leave our armchair to change television channels, but our bodies are still as they were when they were designed for that stone-age world. We were designed for vigorous activity and when we don't get it, our bodies miss it. We're then like badly-tuned engines which don't work efficiently. Even though we consume fewer calories than our forebears, we're not doing enough physical activity to burn up these calories and so we get fat. Increasingly, it's being shown that not having enough exercise is a major – perhaps the main – reason why so many of us are overweight.

'But I've heard,' I can hear you saying, 'that it takes such a lot of exercise to burn off a few calories.' It is true that it would take a three-mile walk to burn off the calories from a large slice of chocolate cake but that is really not the end of the story.

The many ways exercise helps us lose weight

- Over a period of time, even modest amounts of exercise are important. We don't get fat overnight – it's just a few extra calories a day that over the months and years add up to pounds of fat. A small increase in physical activity daily will make an enormous difference over the same period of time. For example, if you walked only an extra mile a day, you'd lose a pound or so each month – about a stone a year.

- In the short term, when we start to take regular exercise to help with our weight loss, our badly-tuned body starts adjusting and gives us weight-reducing benefits out of proportion to the amount of work we put in.

- First of all, exercise does burn off calories. This is more significant than was once supposed. Half-an-hour's walking burns up about 150 calories. But 30×1 minute walks would also burn up 150 calories. Even 60×30 second walks (like walking down the corridor in your office rather than using the phone) would burn up 150 calories. There are, as we'll see, many more benefits to be gained if your exercise is sustained for 20-30 minutes rather than being in short bursts, but at least mini-walks are better than nothing. What you should aim at is some regular sustained exercise; but first, think of all the small ways you can increase your physical activity without your noticing it (there are some ideas for this on pages 165-6).

- Secondly, as we saw in Chapter Three, exercise is important for the effect it has on the 'tickover' speed of our body, the Basal Metabolic Rate (BMR), the energy our body uses up just in keeping us alive. Regular, sustained exercise can cause us to increase our BMR – and this increase continues for several hours after we've stopped exercising. There's evidence that when exercise has become part of our life and our bodies are 'trained' the increased BMR is sustained permanently; this means we're burning up more calories at rest. So we can slim while we sleep! It has to be said that the increase in the BMR is usually quite small, but it is significant. Remember that cutting calories by dieting – on any diet – tends to decrease our BMR. We need the slight increase that regular exercise gives in order to counteract this.

- Next, exercise benefits slimmers by making our bodies efficient at another calorie-cutting activity – thermogenesis. Remember this is the body's ability to burn up excess calories taken in as food energy and produce heat. There's evidence that regular, sustained exercise increases this diet-induced thermogenesis.
- People who don't exercise think that exercise tends to increase the appetite. It doesn't. Most people who exercise regularly find that exercise tends to depress the appetite for an hour or so afterwards. I certainly find this is true. So think of the advantage of exercise before meal-times!
- If you choose the combination of diet and exercise to lose weight, you'll begin to see and feel the benefits before very many pounds have fallen off according to your bathroom scales. Regular exercise has a toning and shaping effect on the body's muscles so you'll feel and look slimmer ahead of that dial pointer on the scales reaching your ideal weight.
- Apart from weight loss, regular exercise will change the ratio of fat and lean tissue in your body – increasing the lean and decreasing the fat, of course! It will cause the percentage of fat to go down from an average of 22 per cent in non-exercising men to 16 per cent in exercising men and from an average of 30 per cent in women who don't exercise to 20 per cent in those who do.
- One further advantage of exercise is that it's something to do other than eating! Going for a walk or mowing the lawn are excellent diversion tactics if you're tempted to eat something you don't need.

The other benefits of exercise As well as all these ways to help you lose weight, regular exercise will give you so many other bonuses.

- it will set you up for the day; you'll feel better, work better and have more energy
- it will help you sleep better and more soundly
- it's a very good way of reducing stress
- it will help keep your joints and muscles in good working order right into old age
- it will strengthen your bones, so that there'll be less risk of osteoporosis, or thinning of the bones, as you grow older
- it will improve your circulation, so that more oxygen will reach all parts of your body
- it will help ensure that your blood pressure remains normal, or help lower it if it is high

- it will help to build up the strength of your heart so it can do its normal work effortlessly and have a bigger reserve capacity
- it will decrease the level of cholesterol in your blood, so making the build-up of fatty deposits in the arteries, which leads to strokes and heart attacks, less likely
- in short, it will help you to become biologically younger than non-exercising people of the same age

How can you resist all these benefits? Anyone can think of several excuses not to exercise, but compared with the benefits, they're all pretty flimsy.

- 'I really am far too fat.' Being overweight really is an excellent reason and incentive to start exercising – it's going to help you to achieve your ideal weight. If you're embarrassed about exercising with other people, there are suggestions later in this chapter for exercises you can do in the privacy of your own bedroom!
- 'I'm too tired.' Regular exercise will help you feel less tired! You'll find you'll have a lot more energy and, sleeping better, will awake refreshed.
- 'I'm too old.' You're never too old to exercise. Of course, as you get older you can't exercise as vigorously, but as long as you're puffing a little, you're getting the maximum benefit. Regular exercise also helps to ensure a more active old age.
- 'I feel fine.' How you feel is a good indication of your health, but it's not the whole story: exercise will help you to *be* healthy. And no matter how well you feel, you'll feel *better* when you exercise regularly.
- 'I'm too busy.' If you're not used to putting aside time to exercise, you may find it difficult to fit into a busy life. But there is exercise *everyone* can take, no matter how busy they are. Also, you may need to assess your priorities: isn't losing weight important to you? Isn't keeping healthy important? Don't think of exercise as a chore; it will become a pleasure, and people who exercise regularly find that they're more relaxed and can cope more easily with work pressures and a busy life.
- 'I'm not sporty.' You don't need to be: there are exercises to suit everyone. Even if you didn't play games at school, you can find an exercise you will enjoy. Exercise doesn't need to be competitive. And even in competitive exercise, you don't have to reach championship level – or anywhere near it – to enjoy a sport and to get benefit from it.

- 'I've heard exercise is dangerous.' Of course, some people will have a heart attack while jogging; but far more will have one lying in bed or sitting watching television, yet these are not considered dangerous pastimes! If a middle-aged person, whose arteries are already partially clogged, suddenly starts taking vigorous exercise, he or she runs an increased risk of a heart attack. But built up gradually, exercise is not only safe, it will also help to protect you against a heart attack and improve your health in so many other ways. Someone who dies jogging might have died even earlier if he hadn't exercised at all.

- 'I've got medical problems.' Most people, even older people, don't need a medical check-up before starting regular exercise. Indeed, some American doctors would say you need a check-up if you don't exercise.

    Obviously, if you're unfit and haven't exercised for a long time, you'd be wise to take it slowly and gently at first. You should consult your doctor first if you've suffered, or are suffering, from any of these conditions, or are worried about any other aspect of your health

    - high blood pressure or heart disease
    - chest problems like asthma or bronchitis
    - back trouble or a slipped disc
    - joint pains or arthritis
    - recuperation from illness or an operation

In all these conditions, the right exercise will help you to be healthier, but it's wise to ask your doctor's advice. If you've got a cold, 'flu, a sore throat or a temperature, it's wise not to exercise until you feel better.

Exercise regularly If you make a plan of how you're going to start increasing your physical activity and then exercising regularly, then you're halfway to succeeding in doing it.

- First, keep an exercise diary for yourself for a couple of days. An example of how one might look is on page 164. You may be really surprised by how little activity you actually undertake in a day.

- After you've looked at your exercise diary, resolve on ten things you're going to do immediately to start increasing the amount of physical activity you undertake in a day. Write them down. The list on pages 165-66 should give some ideas. Each day, consider how well you've done in keeping to them. Keep at these, in *addition* to the exercise you start taking.

EXERCISE DIARY

	Where was I?	What did I do?
7.00- 7.30	In bed	Switched alarm off
7.30- 8.00	In bathroom	Showered, brushed teeth
8.00- 8.30	In bedroom	Dressed; turned over pages of the newspaper
8.30- 9.00	In kitchen	Ate breakfast
9.00- 9.30	In car	Walked 3 yards to car and 10 yards from car to office
9.30-10.00	In office sitting at desk	Telephoned, wrote, walked 20 yards to the loo
10.00-10.30		
10.30-11.00		
11.00-11.30		
11.30-12.00		
12.00-12.30		
12.30- 1.00	Eating sandwiches	Moving hands to mouth!
1.00- 1.30		
1.30- 2.00		
2.00- 2.30	In office sitting at desk	Telephoning, writing, walked 5 yards to another office twice
2.30- 3.00		
3.00- 3.30		
3.30- 4.00		
4.00- 4.30		
4.30- 5.00		
5.30- 6.00	In car	Walked 10 yards from office to car; 3 yards from car to front door
6.00- 6.30	In garden	Sitting
6.30- 7.00		
7.00- 7.30	In kitchen	Eating and drinking – moving hands to mouth!
7.30- 8.00		
8.00- 8.30	In the sitting room	Watching TV – pressing remote control switch!
8.30- 9.00		
9.00- 9.30		
9.30-10.00		
10.00-10.30	In bed	Reading – turning pages
10.30-11.00		
11.00- 7.00	In bed	Asleep – tossing and turning!

- Decide and write down a one- or two-month exercise plan. There are ideas on how to do this below. Think first of all – which exercise am I likely to enjoy and therefore to stick at? Which exercise can I most easily incorporate into my daily routine (and remember the question is 'which exercise' not 'can I incorporate exercise into my daily routine?!'). Am I going to be happy with one exercise or do I need to have several for variety?

- Each week review your exercise plan and what you actually did. If you didn't succeed in fulfulling it, ask yourself why and work out the way you will ensure you fulfil it the next week.

Your exercise plan of action

First, decide if you're fit or unfit.

- If you're under 35 and you've been taking some regular exercise and you can run for a bus without being rendered speechless for five minutes, you can consider that you're fit. If you're over 35 and have been taking regular exercise (2 or 3 times a week) which gets you a little breathless, you can also consider yourself fit.

- If you're over 35 and haven't had any regular exercise recently, consider yourself unfit. If you're under 35 and haven't been out of breath since you left school, then also consider yourself unfit.

Starting moving   If you are very unfit, or it's a long time since you took any form of exercise, you should start by increasing your physical activity gently and gradually before attempting any more vigorous activity. You need to start weaving regular physical activity into your normal life. It's best to think of small ways you can increase your activity in many areas of your life. Sit down and think and you should be able to come up with half a dozen. Write them down, and then any more which come to you later. Check your list every week and tick off the ones that have become a regular part of your life. I'm hoping that you're also going to be taking up some extra regular exercise as well, but these 'little ways of losing weight' will still help and you should keep thinking whether there are any more you could add to your list. Here are a few suggestions.

- walk to work or to the station or at least walk part of the way

- walk to the shops; if you have a lot of shopping to carry back, you could get someone to come and give you a lift
- think before you use your car or get a bus: 'can I walk there?' Walking there and getting a lift or the bus back is a good habit to get into
- get off the bus one or two stops early and walk the rest of the way
- cycle to work or to the shops or just for pleasure!
- use stairs instead of lifts or escalators wherever you can (you burn more calories going *up* stairs, of course)
- do some gardening or some more gardening. Mow the lawn more often (it's good for it and for you!)
- at work, walk if you want to speak to someone in the building; don't use the phone
- walk the dog morning, noon and night if you can – good for him and you!
- keep thinking to yourself 'The more I move, the more calories I'll burn up and the sooner I'll lose weight.'

What sort of exercise?   The best sort of exercise – exercise which is the most efficient at burning up calories and gives us the most health benefits – is aerobic exercise. This is exercise in which we're using the big muscles of the arms and legs rhythmically and we're getting out of puff. Then we're using oxygen from the air, hence aerobic, to release energy from our muscles and so burn up calories. Anaerobic exercise, like weight-lifting and taking part in a tug-of-war, requires short, sharp bursts of energy and uses a different chemical method to get our muscles to work. Although we contract our muscles in anaerobic exercise, we may not be getting out of breath. The very best aerobic exercise for you is the one you enjoy. Aerobic exercise is particularly effective when you're moving your body through space, either on land or in water. Aerobic exercise, as well as burning up calories, tunes up your heart and lungs so that they're stronger and can eventually do the same work with less effort and have a greater reserve capacity.

Some examples of aerobic exercise are
  – brisk walking
  – running or jogging
  – swimming
  – cycling
  – rowing

- tennis (especially singles)
- energetic dancing
- squash
- running on the spot
- climbing stairs
- using a stationary exercise bike
- skipping

To get the most benefit, your exercise needs to be regular and sustained. You can vary the exercise: a couple of days a week you could do half an hour's brisk walking (split into two fifteen minutes if you need to); on another couple of days you could swim for half an hour; on another day you could play tennis for half an hour; on another day you could skip for 10 or 15 minutes – and then you can go for a walk after Sunday lunch! If you do more than this, of course, you'll be getting more benefit for your weight loss programme. For a more detailed exercise plan, see page 171.

If this sounds all too energetic for you, remember that anything is better than nothing. If only one or two sessions of exercise is possible for you, well start there but do try to build it up. Make sure your reasons for not doing more exercise are genuine and not phoney excuses.

To get the maximum benefit for your health, and to ensure you're burning the maximum number of calories, your exercise should be quite vigorous. It should be enough to get you puffing and out of breath. You shouldn't be so out of breath though that you couldn't carry on a conversation if you wanted to. And vigorous exercise shouldn't be uncomfortable or produce pain. We all have a built-in monitor which tells us whether or not we are getting the right amount of exercise for our age and standard of physical fitness: our pulse rate. As you exercise, your heart rate goes up to supply extra oxygen to the muscles (thus burning off extra calories). The rate is a good guide to whether you're exercising vigorously enough or whether you're exercising too strenuously and should slow down. The pulse rate is also a monitor of your fitness: if you're unfit, you'll be able to get your heart rate up to a sufficient speed just by walking.

Take your pulse (on the thumb side of the wrist or at the neck, beside the windpipe) for ten seconds immediately after you've exercised, and multiply it by six (to give the rate for a minute). If your pulse rate is faster than the safe maximum for your age (see table below), you need to take it more easily. If it's below the maximum rate given, you can afford to be more vigorous. You'll soon get to know what's right for you and won't need to keep checking your pulse. If your pulse is irregular, or if you get pain in the chest when you exercise, you should see your doctor.

Check your pulse rate during or immediately after exercise and compare with these figures.

	minimum	maximum
age 20 – 29	140/minute	170/minute
30 – 39	130	160
40 – 49	125	140
50 – 59	115	130
60 – 69	105	120

Now let's look at some of the ways you could use to start shedding those excess pounds.

Walking Remember that walking is one of the very best exercises and is an excellent way to start exercising. It's safe for people of all ages and it can bring you the same benefits as more vigorous forms of exercise provided you do it for long enough and walk fast enough. A casual stroll isn't giving the maximum benefit; you should aim to get out of puff.

But you should build up slowly and aim for a 20 or 30 minute walk where you get out of breath but can still carry on a normal conversation. After a while, you'll want to walk for longer as you'll feel barely warmed up after 20 minutes – so increase the length of time you walk for and try to walk part of the way uphill. Go faster as well.

Even if you start some other form of exercise, you should keep walking as well!

Preparing for more strenuous exercise When you're feeling fitter you'll want to tackle some more vigorous exercise. If you're under 35, you could start with this, but take it slowly and easily at first. Compared with walking, more vigorous exercise will get you fitter faster, and will take less time each day. It will also burn up those calories faster.

Even if you are fit, though, it's always wise to take it slowly for the first five minutes as you warm up. You could start with some gentle bending and stretching exercises. Most injuries and sprains are the result of overdoing it too quickly. Always 'cool down' as well, by walking or moving slowly for a few minutes after you've finished brisk exercise. A lot of blood is sent to your legs to supply them with oxygen during exercise. When your muscles are working hard, the movement helps to shift this blood back to the heart and brain. If you stop suddenly, the blood 'pools' in your legs, your brain doesn't get enough, and you may become dizzy.

After very heavy exercise, you may become dehydrated; it's wise to top up with clear fluids (non-sugary ones) after you've finished, and perhaps during exercise too if it's a hot day and you're sweating a lot.

Running or jogging A jog is really just a slow run. Again, you need to go slowly for several weeks, at first alternating jogging with walking (see chart on page 171). Build up gradually so that you're doing more jogging than walking and then all jogging. Don't get too breathless. You're not in a race, so don't increase your speed until you're ready. The time you spend jogging is more important in burning up calories than the speed at which you jog.

Try to run on grass as it's easier on your feet. You do need to buy a good pair of running shoes: go to a specialist sports shop and ask for advice. You'll get a lot of advice and help too if you join an athletics club. Jogging with a friend of approximately the same standard will encourage you to do it on a regular basis and not to skip it if you don't feel like it on a particular day.

Swimming This is probably the ideal exercise if you are overweight as the water supports the weight of your body. So even if you're very overweight, you should find it easy to swim. It's good for people of all ages and all levels of physical fitness. It's good if you've got joint problems or backache. It's also something you can do with the whole family, so you're more likely to incorporate it into your life permanently. But splashing about with the kids – which is fun for part of the time – doesn't count as aerobic exercise. To burn up those calories, you need to swim laps using one of the serious strokes: crawl, butterfly, backstroke or breaststroke. Build up your stamina so that you reach the point where you can swim for 20 minutes without stopping. If you're conscious about your size, choose a time of the day (like early morning) when not many other people are around.

Cycling Again this may be a pleasant pastime for the whole family, or you could start cycling to work. Cycling is good exercise for those who are overweight, as their body weight is supported. To ensure you get sufficient exercise, get your legs moving hard and rhythmically. Build up gradually and increase the length of time you cycle by five minutes each week. Make sure you know your Highway Code and at night wear reflective clothing.

Badminton, tennis and squash Badminton and tennis can be fun to play even if you're a beginner and again the whole family can join in. You get maximum benefit though as your play improves and you're playing against people of a similar or higher standard. Then the exercise will become more aerobic with fewer stops and starts. Singles tennis is likely to be more vigorous than doubles.

You should already be fit when you start playing squash; it can be a fast, hard game, but it is very efficient at burning off calories. If you're over thirty-five, get fit with some other exercise before you start playing squash, and then begin by playing very gently.

Dancing Waltzing isn't going to burn off too many calories though vigorous disco dancing will. Aerobic dancing classes, however, do provide a way of getting exercise which is of benefit to the heart. Some of them have been criticised for pushing people too quickly and so causing injuries or sprains, but some people enjoy exercising in company and find it encourages them to keep going. If you begin gradually, it's a good way of getting exercise.

Keep-fit classes and work-outs If you want to do work-outs – bending and stretching exercise – you'll find that by far the best way of keeping at it is by going to keep-fit classes. It can get rather boring on your own. Some keep-fit classes are run especially for people who are overweight.

Make sure that you're getting reasonably breathless though – gently waving your arms around doesn't count as aerobic exercise! With this sort of keep-fit group, you burn off more calories walking briskly there and back home!

Indoor activities If you don't want to exercise in public, you can burn off those calories in the privacy of your own home. Most

SUGGESTIONS FOR AN EXERCISE PLAN Try to do one session five days a week.

		WEEK 1	WEEK 2	WEEK 3	WEEK 4	WEEK 5	WEEK 6
Brisk Walking	Unfit	5	10	15	20	25	30
	Fit	10	20	25	25	30	35
Swimming	Unfit	5	10	15	20	25	30
	Fit	10	15	20	25	30	35
Skipping	Unfit	3	4	5	6	7	8
	Fit	2 x 5	10	2 x 6	15	2 x 9	20
Rowing & Cycling Machine	Unfit	5	7	10	12	15	20
	Fit	10	12	15	20	25	30
Aerobics Dancing	Unfit	5	8	10	12	15	20
	Fit	20	25	30	40	50	60
Cycling	Unfit	5	7	10	15	20	25
	Fit	15	20	25	30	35	40
Jogging	Unfit	Don't jog – 5 brisk walking	5 Alternate 15 secs jogging & 15 secs brisk walking	10 Alternate 30 secs jogging & 30 secs brisk walking	15 Alternate 1 min jogging & 1 min brisk walking	20 Alternate 2 mins jogging & 2 mins brisk walking	25 Alternate 5 mins jogging & 5 mins brisk walking
	Fit	10 Alternate 10 secs jogging & 10 secs brisk walking	15 Alternate 30 secs jogging & 30 secs brisk walking	20 Alternate 1 min jogging & 1 min brisk walking	5 mins brisk walking 10 mins jogging 5 mins brisk walking	5 mins brisk walking 15 mins jogging 5 mins brisk walking	20 mins jogging

MINUTES PER SESSION

of these solitary activities are rather boring and repetitive but you can always listen to music or the radio at the same time, have a conversation, or even watch television.

– skipping with a rope is superb aerobic exercise. Ten minutes quick skipping burns up 100 calories! It is very strenuous and you should start gently.

– running on the spot will also provide good exercise but is rather more boring

– repeatedly going up and down stairs is good aerobic exercise – but you need to check your pulse rate with this as it's an exercise which will rapidly increase your heart rate

– stationary bikes and rowing machines will give you excellent exercise. The very cheap ones are rather flimsy, so spend a bit more money – that will encourage you to use the thing as well! The best kinds of exercise bikes have adjustable pedal resistance so that you can work harder as you get fitter. Be sure you're really going to use one before you buy.

Apart from being private, all these activities are useful if you have a busy life and can't see where exercise would fit in.

Keep at it

Even when you've reached your ideal weight – keep exercising. You can ring the changes so you don't get bored. Keeping exercising is your best insurance policy against regaining weight. You'll also be staying fit and healthy. Fitness isn't something you put into a deposit account and draw out when you need it. You need to earn it, week by week. But once you start to exercise regularly, you'll feel so much better and enjoy life so much that you'll wonder why you didn't always do it.

CHAPTER 9

SLIMMING IN SPECIAL CASES

In general, whoever you are, you can lose weight in the same way: the BBC Diet is healthy for everyone. But at particular stages of life there are some special considerations and this chapter highlights the important points about slimming in childhood and adolescence; pregnancy and after childbirth; the menopause and old age.

SLIMMING AND CHILDREN

You should be concerned that your baby doesn't get fat; one of the best ways to ensure this is to breast feed. Bottle-fed babies are more likely to get overweight than breast-fed ones. If your baby is fat, discuss what you can do with your health visitor.

Remember that there's an increased risk that overweight children will become overweight adults. So we should take overweight children seriously; it's not justified just to assume that fat children will 'grow out of it'. Certainly it seems that the majority will; but a sizeable number will become fat adults.

It seems that often, the very obese people who need to be treated for their overweight at hospital clinics begin to become overweight when they are children. Remember that if you or your spouse are overweight (and particularly if you both are) then your children are more likely to become overweight. It's not inevitable, but you should try to do something about it before it happens.

It's very useful to get your child to fill in a food diary (see page 56) – you could make it fun and treat it as a game. Pay particular attention to what's eaten at school meals and at break-times. Then what you need to be doing is changing the diet of the whole family to a more healthy and less fattening one. This will have benefits for you as well, but it will have particular benefits for your children. If your child is overweight, you need to think in the same way as you would for yourself: how can I reduce fat and sugar in his or her diet and how can I increase the fibre? It's unfair to expect a child to change his or her eating habits when the rest of the family don't – this is an ideal opportunity for the whole family to switch to a healthier diet.

The problem of overweight in children is more complicated than in adults because weight gain does depend partly on height gain. It is important to determine whether the child's pattern of eating or exercise is unusual. It's advisable therefore to take your doctor's advice. Remember that the principles outlined in the BBC Diet apply to children as much as adults. The one thing that should be mentioned is that children under two derive many of their calories from milk; it's wise to give them whole milk until this age and then get them used to semi-skimmed and then skimmed milk.

SLIMMING AND ADOLESCENTS

Attempts to slim obese young teenagers have sometimes been discouraged because it was thought that the development of anorexia nervosa would be encouraged, particularly in girls. But anorexia is not caused by slimming and there is certainly no reason not to encourage teenagers – overweight or not – to follow a healthy and therefore non-fattening eating pattern.

Anorexia nervosa occurs in about 1 per cent of girls aged 16–18 years and is very uncommon, though not unknown, in boys. It's really a distortion of body image, coupled with, it's thought, a rejection of the process of sexual maturity. Those who suffer from anorexia may be of normal weight or even thin, but think that they are fat and need to lose weight.

Anorexia nervosa needs specialist medical treatment, but remember it's not a reason for the teenager who is actually overweight stopping losing weight.

SLIMMING IN PREGANCY AND AFTER CHILDBIRTH

The average weight gain in pregnancy is about 27 lb (12.5 kg). About 15 lb (7 kg) of this is water; 2 lb (1 kg) is protein of which half is in the baby; and about 10 lb (4 kg) of fat is added to the mother's energy stores as a reserve to support the supply of milk during breast-feeding. In pregnancy especially the quality of the food, and not its quantity, is important. There appears to be a small increase in food intake in early pregnancy and little change thereafter. There's a fall in physical activity in late pregnancy. In addition, it seems an alteration in metabolic efficiency occurs, which enables the extra fat to be laid down despite the increasing needs of the baby.

The total energy cost of pregnancy and breast-feeding has been calculated at 80 800 calories! It's certainly been shown that the baby is not at a disadvantage, and indeed may be at an advantage, if the mother gains less weight than 27 lbs (12.5 kg). Indeed, most doctors believe that a weight gain of about 15 lb (7 kg) overall would be most beneficial for the baby and, in this case, the mother's weight after delivery would be less than before pregnancy. Against this must be set the other known fact that there's a possibility of the growth of the baby being affected if the mother is malnourished.

This is quite unlikely in this country if the mother begins her pregnancy healthy and well-nourished. In fact, compared with the young of other species, the human baby is quite small and slow-growing and so isn't a great nutritional burden to the mother.

So what conclusion can one come to? Obviously, you're going to be attending ante-natal clinics and taking your doctor's advice. If you are overweight, pregnancy may be an opportunity to control your weight. Talk to your doctor about it. Certainly you can follow the guidelines of the BBC Diet, but don't restrict the quantity of the food you eat. (You'll probably find it difficult to restrict anyway, as during pregnancy the appetite increases.) If you're eating the quantity you wish, but cutting down fatty and sugary food and increasing food rich in fibre, you should end your pregnancy weighing less than before you became pregnant.

There is a tendency for women to become fatter with increasing age, but the number of children you have, on the whole, makes only a negligible contribution to this weight increase. This is true for most women, though there are some, who are already the most overweight, for whom pregnancy is associated with a much greater weight gain.

When you're breast feeding, the energy required to produce the milk each day comes to about 675 calories. This energy is normally supplied by breaking down the extra 10 lb (4 kg) or so of fat which have been laid down during pregnancy. This is another good reason for breast feeding – you're helping yourself and your baby not to get fat.

Even if food has been restricted during pregnancy, this doesn't seem to affect lactation. Again, following the guidelines of the BBC Diet is perfectly safe when you're breastfeeding. Certainly 'eating for two' is no excuse to eat excessively – one of the two is very tiny!

SLIMMING AND THE MENOPAUSE

Sex hormones do certainly influence the amount of fat in the body, as evidenced by the differences in body fat between men and women. Women who have had their ovaries removed (usually as part of a hysterectomy) frequently tend to put on weight.

In the United Kingdom, women as a group tend to put on weight around the time of the menopause, but whether this is because of metabolic, physiological or social reasons is unclear.

Whatever the reason, you need to be particularly careful about watching your weight around the time of the menopause. You can safely and healthily follow all the recommendations of the BBC Diet.

SLIMMING AND OLDER PEOPLE

We seem to have accepted in Britain that it's normal to put on weight as we get older. It's certainly common but it isn't normal. There's no need to put on extra weight as we get older and there's every reason to make sure we don't – we'll feel better and be more mobile for one thing. How you look becomes less important as you get older and even how long you live becomes less important – what becomes increasingly important is the quality of life you have. If you're fat, your quality of life will certainly be improved if you lose weight.

You can follow the BBC Diet no matter how old you are. And remember you can – and should – take some exercise no matter what your age is. Look at Chapter Eight to see all the benefits exercise brings no matter what your age.

LIST OF RECIPES

BBC COOKERY BOOKS

Sarah Brown's
New Vegetarian Kitchen

Sarah Brown introduced the basic principles of vegetarian cookery to a wide and appreciative audience through the highly successful BBC-tv series *Vegetarian Kitchen* and the bestselling book she wrote to accompany the programmes. Since then, a growing number of people have fundamentally changed their eating habits, and many more are incorporating vegetarian dishes into their diet on a regular basis.

Now Sarah Brown offers advice, encouragement and inspiration for all those who are ready to move a stage further. Beginning with a helpful chapter on creating vegetarian meals, she provides 150 tempting new recipes – from soups, pâtés and snacks to salads, breads, cakes and puddings – including plenty of main course ideas based on pasta, grains, pancakes, casseroles and bakes. Building from basic 'blueprint' recipes, she expands the range of ingredients and techniques to widen the scope for individual creativity and expertise. With additional hints on microwave cooking, freezing, choosing wines and cooking for children, Sarah Brown's *New Vegetarian Kitchen* will be warmly welcomed by everyone interested in vegetarian cuisine.

The Fish Course

Fresh fish is back on top! That's the message from Susan Hicks, cookery writer and presenter of the BBC's cookery series, *The Fish Course*. After years of neglect it is once more being recognised as a particularly healthy and nutritious part of our diet, and here she demonstrates in over 150 recipes how versatile and delicious it is too.

First of all, Susan explains how to cook each fish *perfectly* and then enhance its natural taste and texture with the lightest of sauces and subtlest of flavourings. Her innovative combinations are both mouthwatering and simple to put together – try baked trout with oranges and thyme, for example, or fish and fennel risotto, or baked bass with sorrel sauce. Microwave cooking instructions are given wherever appropriate, and as well as the many recipes for family meals and classic dishes for entertaining, Susan also suggests some ways of combining fish with unusual ingredients such as sea vegetables. Her advice on what to look for when shopping for fish, the illustrated step-by-step guides to preparing what you select and a comprehensive glossary make this both a stimulating collection of recipes and an indispensable handbook to the art of fish cookery.

Floyd on Fish

A witty, informative and entertaining book about cooking and eating fish that will inspire the enthusiastic beginner and delight more experienced cooks. There's advice on how to recognise, handle, and clean the fish, on the sauces and butters to serve with them – and a whole wealth of classic and original recipes, including some of the great fish dishes of the world, like Bouillabaisse, Paella, Sashimi and Teppanyaki, as well as beautifully simple ideas – what easier than to charcoal grill fresh pilchards or sardines over a barbecue in your garden? – and new and exciting combinations of flavour and texture. Ever since he caught his first trout as a boy, Keith Floyd has been passionate about fish, and his love and knowledge of the subject – accumulated over the years as a restaurateur in France and England, and now as a writer and television presenter – is evident on every page. A book to enjoy, preferably with a glass of wine to hand, and a book, above all, to use.